2. Lentil and vegetable soup

Ingredients:

• 1 cup brown or green lentils, rinsed
• 6 cups low•sodium vegetable or chicken broth
• 1 tbsp olive oil
• 1 onion, diced
• 3 carrots, peeled and diced
• 3 celery stalks, diced
• 3 garlic cloves, minced
• 1 tsp ground cumin
• 1 tsp dried thyme
• Salt and pepper to taste
• Chopped parsley for garnish (optional)

Instructions:

1. In a large pot, bring the lentils and broth to a boil over high heat. Reduce heat to medium•low, cover, and simmer for 20•25 minutes, until the lentils are tender.

2. In a separate skillet, heat the olive oil over medium heat. Add the onion, carrots, and celery. Sauté for 5•7 minutes, until the vegetables are softened.

3. Add the garlic, cumin, and thyme to the skillet. Cook for 1 minute, until fragrant.

4. Transfer the sautéed vegetables to the pot with the cooked lentils. Stir to combine.

5. Season the soup with salt and pepper to taste. Serve the lentil and vegetable soup hot, garnished with chopped parsley if desired.

This soup is suitable for a fatty liver diet for seniors for the following reasons:

• Lentils are a great source of plant•based protein, fiber, and complex carbohydrates, which can help support liver health.
• The vegetables, such as carrots, celery, and onions, provide a variety of vitamins, minerals, and antioxidants.
• The use of low•sodium broth and minimal added salt helps to limit sodium intake, which is important for those with fatty liver disease.
• The soup is a low•calorie, nutrient•dense meal that can be easily adjusted to meet individual dietary needs.

As always, it's best to consult with a healthcare professional for personalized dietary recommendations for seniors with fatty liver disease.

3. Quinoa salad with chickpeas, tomatoes, and cucumbers

Ingredients:

• 1 cup uncooked quinoa, rinsed
• 1 (15 oz) can chickpeas, drained and rinsed
• 1 cup cherry tomatoes, halved
• 1 cucumber, diced
• 1/2 red onion, thinly sliced
• 2 tbsp olive oil
• 2 tbsp lemon juice
• 1 tsp Dijon mustard
• 1 garlic clove, minced
• 1/4 cup chopped fresh parsley
• Salt and pepper to taste

Instructions:

1. Cook the quinoa according to package instructions. Allow to cool completely.

2. In a large bowl, combine the cooked quinoa, chickpeas, cherry tomatoes, cucumber, and red onion.

3. In a small bowl, whisk together the olive oil, lemon juice, Dijon mustard, and garlic.

4. Pour the dressing over the quinoa salad and toss to coat evenly.

5. Stir in the chopped parsley and season with salt and pepper to taste.

6. Serve chilled or at room temperature.

This quinoa salad is suitable for a fatty liver diet for seniors for the following reasons:

• Quinoa is a gluten•free, high•protein grain that is rich in fiber, vitamins, and minerals.
• Chickpeas are a good source of plant•based protein, fiber, and complex carbohydrates.
• Tomatoes and cucumbers provide a variety of antioxidants, vitamins, and minerals.
• The olive oil and lemon juice•based dressing is a healthy fat source.
• The dish is low in sodium and can be easily adjusted to meet individual dietary needs.

This salad can be a nutritious and filling meal or side dish for seniors with fatty liver disease. As always, it's best to consult with a healthcare professional for personalized dietary recommendations.

Welcome to the ***"Fatty Liver Diet Cookbook for Seniors: 110+ Nourishing and Satisfying Meals for Optimal Liver Health."*** As we age, our bodies undergo numerous changes, and maintaining our health becomes increasingly crucial. One of the key aspects of good health is ensuring our liver functions optimally. This cookbook is specifically designed to help seniors manage and improve their liver health through delicious, easy-to-prepare meals.

Fatty liver disease, also known as hepatic steatosis, affects millions of people worldwide. It occurs when excess fat builds up in the liver, potentially leading to serious health issues. However, with the right diet and lifestyle changes, it is possible to manage and even reverse the effects of fatty liver disease. This book provides a comprehensive collection of recipes that are not only tasty but also tailored to support liver health.

Why a Fatty Liver Diet?
A fatty liver diet focuses on reducing fat intake, increasing fiber, and incorporating essential nutrients that promote liver function. This diet emphasizes whole grains, lean proteins, healthy fats, fruits, and vegetables while avoiding processed foods, excessive sugars, and unhealthy fats. By following this diet, you can help reduce liver inflammation, improve liver function, and support overall well-being.

Why is this Cookbook for Seniors?
As seniors, our nutritional needs change, and it's important to consume foods that cater to these needs. This cookbook takes into consideration the dietary requirements and potential health concerns of seniors, offering recipes that are easy to digest, nutrient-rich, and simple to prepare. Whether you're cooking for yourself or a loved one, these recipes are designed to make healthy eating enjoyable and manageable.

What to Expect?
In this cookbook, you'll find over 110 carefully curated recipes that cater to breakfast, lunch, dinner, and snacks. Each recipe is crafted to be liver-friendly, delicious, and easy to follow. From hearty breakfasts to satisfying dinners and delightful desserts, there's something for every taste and occasion. Additionally, the recipes come with nutritional information to help you keep track of your dietary intake and ensure you're meeting your health goals.

Beyond recipes, this book also offers valuable tips on meal planning, grocery shopping, and understanding the nutritional aspects of a fatty liver diet. You'll learn about the best foods to include in your diet, how to prepare them in a way that maximizes their health benefits, and strategies to maintain a balanced and enjoyable eating routine.

Embark on a journey to better liver health with these nourishing and satisfying meals. Whether you're new to the fatty liver diet or looking to expand your culinary repertoire, this cookbook is your trusted companion in the kitchen. Let's take the first step towards a healthier, happier you.

1. Grilled salmon with roasted asparagus

Ingredients:

• 4 salmon fillets (about 4•6 oz each)
• 1 lb asparagus, trimmed
• 2 tbsp olive oil
• Salt and pepper to taste
• Lemon wedges for serving

Instructions:
1. Preheat grill or grill pan to medium•high heat.

2. Toss the asparagus with 1 tbsp of olive oil and season with salt and pepper.

3. Arrange the asparagus in a single layer on a baking sheet. Roast in the preheated oven for 12•15 minutes, until tender and lightly browned.

4. Brush the salmon fillets with the remaining 1 tbsp of olive oil and season with salt and pepper.

5. Grill the salmon for 4•6 minutes per side, or until it flakes easily with a fork and reaches an internal temperature of 145°F.

6. Serve the grilled salmon immediately with the roasted asparagus and lemon wedges.

This recipe is suitable for a fatty liver diet for seniors for a few reasons:

• Salmon is an excellent source of omega•3 fatty acids, which can help reduce inflammation and support liver health.
• Asparagus is a nutrient•dense vegetable that is low in calories and high in fiber, vitamins, and minerals.
• The dish is baked and grilled, which are healthier cooking methods compared to frying.
• The use of olive oil provides healthy monounsaturated fats.

Be sure to adjust portion sizes as needed to meet the individual's caloric and nutritional needs. Consult with a healthcare professional for personalized dietary recommendations.

4. Turkey and avocado wrap in whole wheat tortilla

Ingredients:

• 4 whole wheat tortillas
• 8 oz sliced turkey breast
• 1 avocado, sliced
• 1 cup baby spinach or arugula
• 2 tbsp hummus
• 1 tbsp olive oil
• 1 tbsp lemon juice
• Salt and pepper to taste

Instructions:
1. In a small bowl, mix together the olive oil and lemon juice to make a simple dressing.

2. Lay the whole wheat tortillas on a flat surface. Spread 1/2 tbsp of hummus on each tortilla.

3. Arrange the sliced turkey, avocado, and spinach or arugula on the tortillas.

4. Drizzle the olive oil and lemon dressing over the fillings.

5. Season with salt and pepper to taste.

6. Carefully roll up the tortillas, tucking in the sides as you go. Cut the wraps in half diagonally and serve.

This turkey and avocado wrap is suitable for a fatty liver diet for seniors for the following reasons:

• Whole wheat tortillas provide complex carbohydrates, fiber, and B vitamins.
• Turkey is a lean protein source that is low in saturated fat.
• Avocado is a healthy source of monounsaturated fats, which can help reduce inflammation.
• Spinach or arugula adds additional vitamins, minerals, and antioxidants.
• Hummus provides plant•based protein and fiber.
• The olive oil and lemon dressing is a simple, healthy fat source.

This wrap can be a satisfying and nutrient•dense meal or snack for seniors with fatty liver disease. As always, it's best to consult with a healthcare professional for personalized dietary recommendations.

5. Baked sweet potato with steamed broccoli

Ingredients:

• 2 medium sweet potatoes, scrubbed clean
• 1 lb broccoli florets
• 1 tbsp olive oil
• Salt and pepper to taste

Instructions:
1. Preheat the oven to 400°F.

2. Pierce the sweet potatoes several times with a fork. Place them directly on the oven rack and bake for 45•60 minutes, or until they are tender when pierced with a fork.

3. While the sweet potatoes are baking, prepare the broccoli. Fill a medium saucepan with about 1 inch of water and bring it to a boil. Add the broccoli florets, cover, and steam for 5•7 minutes, until the broccoli is tender but still bright green.

4. Drain the broccoli and transfer it to a serving bowl. Drizzle with the olive oil and season with salt and pepper to taste.

5. Once the sweet potatoes are cooked, remove them from the oven and let them cool for a few minutes. Slice them open and serve with the steamed broccoli.

This baked sweet potato and steamed broccoli dish is suitable for a fatty liver diet for seniors for the following reasons:

• Sweet potatoes are a nutrient•dense carbohydrate source that is high in fiber, vitamins, and antioxidants.

• Broccoli is a cruciferous vegetable that is low in calories and high in fiber, vitamins, and minerals.

• The dish is baked and steamed, which are healthier cooking methods compared to frying.

• The use of olive oil provides a healthy source of monounsaturated fats. The meal is low in sodium and can be easily adjusted to meet individual dietary needs.

This simple and nutritious dish can be a great option for seniors with fatty liver disease. As always, it's best to consult with a healthcare professional for personalized dietary recommendations.

6. Grilled chicken with roasted zucchini and bell peppers

Ingredients:

• 4 boneless, skinless chicken breasts
• 2 zucchini, sliced into 1/2•inch rounds
• 2 bell peppers (any color), sliced into 1•inch pieces
• 2 tbsp olive oil
• 1 tsp dried oregano
• 1 tsp garlic powder
• Salt and pepper to taste

Instructions:

1. Preheat the grill or grill pan to medium•high heat.

2. In a large bowl, toss the zucchini and bell pepper slices with 1 tbsp of the olive oil, oregano, garlic powder, salt, and pepper.

3. Spread the vegetables in a single layer on a baking sheet. Roast in the preheated oven for 15•20 minutes, flipping halfway, until tender and lightly charred.

4. Brush the chicken breasts with the remaining 1 tbsp of olive oil and season with salt and pepper.

5. Grill the chicken for 4•6 minutes per side, or until it reaches an internal temperature of 165°F. Serve the grilled chicken immediately with the roasted zucchini and bell peppers.

This grilled chicken and roasted vegetable dish is suitable for a fatty liver diet for seniors for the following reasons:

• Chicken is a lean protein source that is low in saturated fat.
• Zucchini and bell peppers are low•calorie, nutrient•dense vegetables that are high in fiber, vitamins, and antioxidants.
• The dish is grilled and roasted, which are healthier cooking methods compared to frying.
• The use of olive oil provides a healthy source of monounsaturated fats.
• The meal is low in sodium and can be easily adjusted to meet individual dietary needs.

This simple and flavorful dish can be a great option for seniors with fatty liver disease. As always, it's best to consult with a healthcare professional for personalized dietary recommendations.

7. Baked cod with sautéed spinach

Ingredients:

• 4 cod fillets (about 4•6 oz each)
• 2 tbsp olive oil
• 2 garlic cloves, minced
• 5 oz baby spinach
• 1 tbsp lemon juice
• Salt and pepper to taste

Instructions:

1. Preheat the oven to 400°F.

2. Place the cod fillets in a baking dish and season with salt and pepper.

3. Bake the cod for 12•15 minutes, or until it flakes easily with a fork and reaches an internal temperature of 145°F.

4. While the cod is baking, heat the olive oil in a large skillet over medium heat. Add the minced garlic and sauté for 1 minute, until fragrant.

5. Add the baby spinach to the skillet and sauté for 2•3 minutes, until the spinach is wilted.

6. Remove the skillet from the heat and stir in the lemon juice. Season the sautéed spinach with salt and pepper to taste. Serve the baked cod immediately, topped with the sautéed spinach.

This baked cod and sautéed spinach dish is suitable for a fatty liver diet for seniors for the following reasons:

• Cod is a lean, low•mercury fish that is high in protein and omega•3 fatty acids, which can help support liver health.
• Spinach is a nutrient•dense leafy green that is high in vitamins, minerals, and antioxidants.
• The dish is baked and sautéed, which are healthier cooking methods compared to frying.
• The use of olive oil provides a healthy source of monounsaturated fats.
• The meal is low in sodium and can be easily adjusted to meet individual dietary needs.

This simple and flavorful dish can be a great option for seniors with fatty liver disease. As always, it's best to consult with a healthcare professional for personalized dietary recommendations.

8. Vegetable stir•fry with tofu

Ingredients:

• 1 block (14 oz) firm or
extra•firm tofu, cubed
• 2 tbsp low•sodium soy sauce or tamari
• 1 tbsp sesame oil
• 2 tbsp olive oil
• 3 cloves garlic, minced

• 1 inch piece fresh ginger, peeled and grated
• 1 red bell pepper, sliced
• 1 cup broccoli florets
• 1 cup sliced mushrooms
• 1 cup snow peas or snap peas
• 2 cups baby spinach
• 1 tbsp rice vinegar
• Salt and pepper to taste
• Cooked brown rice, for serving (optional)

Instructions:

1. In a medium bowl, toss the cubed tofu with the soy sauce or tamari and 1 tbsp of the sesame oil. Set aside.

2. Heat the remaining 1 tbsp of olive oil in a large skillet or wok over medium•high heat. Add the garlic and ginger and sauté for 1 minute, until fragrant.

3. Add the bell pepper, broccoli, mushrooms, and snow peas to the skillet. Stir•fry for 4•5 minutes, until the vegetables are tender•crisp.

4. Add the marinated tofu and the baby spinach to the skillet. Stir•fry for an additional 2•3 minutes, until the spinach is wilted.

5. Remove the skillet from the heat and stir in the rice vinegar. Season with salt and pepper to taste. Serve the vegetable stir•fry immediately, over cooked brown rice if desired.

This vegetable stir•fry with tofu is suitable for a fatty liver diet for seniors for the following reasons:

• Tofu is a plant•based protein source that is low in saturated fat.
• The variety of vegetables, such as bell peppers, broccoli, mushrooms, and spinach, provide a wide range of vitamins, minerals, and antioxidants.
• The dish is stir•fried, which is a healthy cooking method that preserves the nutrients in the vegetables.
• The use of low•sodium soy sauce or tamari and minimal added salt helps to limit sodium intake.
• The meal is low in calories and can be easily adjusted to meet individual dietary needs.

This flavorful and nutrient•dense stir•fry can be a great option for seniors with fatty liver disease. As always, it's best to consult with a healthcare professional for personalized dietary recommendations.

9. Lentil and vegetable curry

Ingredients:

- 1 cup brown or green lentils, rinsed
- 4 cups low•sodium vegetable broth
- 1 tbsp olive oil
- 1 onion, diced
- 3 cloves garlic, minced
- 1 tbsp grated fresh ginger
- 1 tsp ground cumin
- 1 tsp ground coriander
- 1 tsp garam masala
- 1/2 tsp turmeric
- 1 cup diced tomatoes (fresh or canned)
- 1 cup diced cauliflower
- 1 cup diced sweet potato
- 1 cup frozen peas
- 1/4 cup chopped fresh cilantro
- Salt and pepper to taste
- Cooked brown rice, for serving (optional)

Instructions:

1. In a large pot, combine the lentils and vegetable broth. Bring to a boil, then reduce heat and simmer for 20•25 minutes, until the lentils are tender.

2. In a separate skillet, heat the olive oil over medium heat. Add the onion and sauté for 3•4 minutes, until translucent.

3. Add the garlic, ginger, cumin, coriander, garam masala, and turmeric to the skillet. Cook for 1 minute, until fragrant.

4. Stir the diced tomatoes, cauliflower, sweet potato, and frozen peas into the skillet. Cook for 8•10 minutes, until the vegetables are tender.

5. Add the cooked lentils and their cooking liquid to the skillet. Stir to combine and simmer for an additional 5 minutes.

6. Remove from heat and stir in the chopped cilantro. Season with salt and pepper to taste. Serve the lentil and vegetable curry over cooked brown rice, if desired.

This lentil and vegetable curry is suitable for a fatty liver diet for seniors for the following reasons:

- Lentils are a great source of plant•based protein, fiber, and complex carbohydrates.
- The variety of vegetables, such as cauliflower, sweet potato, and peas, provide a wide range of vitamins, minerals, and antioxidants.
- The use of low•sodium vegetable broth and minimal added salt helps to limit sodium intake.
- The dish is simmered, which is a healthy cooking method that preserves the nutrients in the ingredients.
- The meal is low in calories and can be easily adjusted to meet individual dietary needs.

10. Whole wheat pasta with marinara sauce and grilled vegetables

Ingredients:

• 8 oz whole wheat pasta
• 1 tbsp olive oil
• 1 eggplant, sliced into 1/2•inch rounds
• 1 zucchini, sliced into 1/2•inch rounds
• 1 red bell pepper, sliced into strips
• 1 onion, sliced into 1/2•inch rings
• 2 cups marinara sauce (low•sodium if possible)
• 2 tbsp grated Parmesan cheese (optional)
• Fresh basil leaves for garnish (optional)

Instructions:

1. Preheat the grill or grill pan to medium•high heat. Bring a large pot of salted water to a boil. Cook the whole wheat pasta according to package instructions, then drain and set aside.

2. Brush the eggplant, zucchini, bell pepper, and onion slices with the olive oil. Season with salt and pepper.

3. Grill the vegetables for 3•4 minutes per side, or until they are tender and have grill marks. Remove the grilled vegetables from the grill and slice or chop them into bite•sized pieces.

4. In a large bowl, toss the cooked whole wheat pasta with the marinara sauce and the grilled vegetables. Serve the pasta and vegetable mixture warm, garnished with grated Parmesan cheese and fresh basil leaves if desired.

This whole wheat pasta dish with grilled vegetables is suitable for a fatty liver diet for seniors for the following reasons:

• Whole wheat pasta provides complex carbohydrates, fiber, and B vitamins.
• The variety of grilled vegetables, such as eggplant, zucchini, bell pepper, and onion, are low in calories and high in fiber, vitamins, and antioxidants.
• The use of a low•sodium marinara sauce helps to limit sodium intake.
• The dish is grilled, which is a healthier cooking method compared to frying.
• The optional Parmesan cheese provides a small amount of healthy fat and protein.

This colorful and flavorful pasta dish can be a great option for seniors with fatty liver disease. As always, it's best to consult with a healthcare professional for personalized dietary recommendations.

11. Oatmeal with fresh berries and almonds

Ingredients:

• 1 cup old•fashioned oats
• 2 cups low•fat or unsweetened almond milk
• 1/4 tsp ground cinnamon
• 1 cup fresh berries (such as blueberries, raspberries, or strawberries)
• 2 tbsp sliced almonds
• 1 tsp honey (optional)

Instructions:

1. In a medium saucepan, combine the oats and almond milk. Bring to a simmer over medium heat, stirring occasionally.

2. Reduce the heat to low and continue to cook the oatmeal, stirring frequently, for 5•7 minutes, or until it reaches your desired consistency.

3. Remove the oatmeal from the heat and stir in the ground cinnamon.

4. Transfer the oatmeal to serving bowls and top with the fresh berries and sliced almonds.

5. Drizzle with a small amount of honey if desired.

This oatmeal with fresh berries and almonds is suitable for a fatty liver diet for seniors for the following reasons:

• Oats are a whole grain that are high in fiber, which can help support liver health.
• Berries are low in calories and high in antioxidants, vitamins, and minerals.
• Almonds are a source of healthy fats, protein, and fiber.
• The dish is low in added sugars, as the honey is optional.
• The use of low•fat or unsweetened almond milk helps to limit saturated fat and added sugars.

This breakfast dish is a nutritious and filling option for seniors with fatty liver disease. The combination of complex carbohydrates, fiber, protein, and healthy fats can help support overall liver function and general health.

As always, it's best to consult with a healthcare professional for personalized dietary recommendations.

12. Egg white omelet with mushrooms and spinach

Ingredients:

• 4 egg whites
• 1 tbsp olive oil
• 1 cup sliced mushrooms
• 1 cup fresh spinach leaves
• 1 tbsp grated Parmesan cheese (optional)
• Salt and pepper to taste

Instructions:

1. In a small bowl, whisk the egg whites until they are light and frothy.

2. Heat the olive oil in a non•stick skillet over medium heat.

3. Add the sliced mushrooms to the skillet and sauté for 3•4 minutes, until they are tender.

4. Add the fresh spinach leaves to the skillet and sauté for an additional 1•2 minutes, until the spinach is wilted.

5. Pour the whisked egg whites into the skillet, covering the mushrooms and spinach.

6. Cook the omelet for 2•3 minutes, until the bottom is set.

7. Carefully flip the omelet and cook for an additional 1•2 minutes, until the egg is fully cooked.

8. Slide the omelet onto a plate and top with the grated Parmesan cheese, if desired.

9. Season the omelet with salt and pepper to taste.

This egg white omelet with mushrooms and spinach is suitable for a fatty liver diet for seniors for the following reasons:

• Egg whites are a lean protein source that are low in cholesterol and saturated fat.
• Mushrooms and spinach are nutrient•dense vegetables that are high in fiber, vitamins, and antioxidants.
• The use of olive oil provides a healthy source of monounsaturated fats.
• The optional Parmesan cheese adds a small amount of healthy fat and protein.
• The dish is low in calories and can be easily adjusted to meet individual dietary needs.

13. Greek yogurt with fresh fruits

Ingredients:

• 1 cup plain Greek yogurt
• 1 cup mixed fresh fruits (such as berries, sliced peaches, or diced mango)
• 1 tbsp honey (optional)
• 1 tbsp chopped walnuts or almonds (optional)

Instructions:
1. In a serving bowl, place the plain Greek yogurt.

2. Top the yogurt with the mixed fresh fruits.

3. If desired, drizzle the honey over the fruit and yogurt.

4. Sprinkle the chopped walnuts or almonds over the top.

This Greek yogurt with fresh fruits is suitable for a fatty liver diet for seniors for the following reasons:

• Greek yogurt is a high•protein, low•fat dairy product that can help support liver health.

• Fresh fruits, such as berries, peaches, and mango, are low in calories and high in fiber, vitamins, and antioxidants.

• The optional honey provides a natural sweetener, which can help satisfy a sweet craving without added sugars.

• The optional nuts, such as walnuts or almonds, add a source of healthy fats and protein.

• The dish is low in sodium and can be easily adjusted to meet individual dietary needs.

This simple and nutritious breakfast or snack can be a great option for seniors with fatty liver disease. The combination of protein, fiber, and healthy fats can help promote feelings of fullness and support overall liver function.

14. Avocado toast on whole grain bread

Ingredients:

• 2 slices of whole grain bread
• 1 ripe avocado, mashed
• 1 tbsp olive oil
• 1 tbsp lemon juice
• 1/4 tsp garlic powder
• Salt and pepper to taste
• Optional toppings: sliced tomatoes, sliced radishes, crumbled feta cheese, chopped fresh herbs

Instructions:

1. Toast the whole grain bread until lightly golden brown.

2. In a small bowl, mash the avocado with the olive oil, lemon juice, and garlic powder. Season with salt and pepper to taste.

3. Spread the mashed avocado mixture evenly over the toasted whole grain bread slices.

4. If desired, top the avocado toast with any of the optional toppings, such as sliced tomatoes, radishes, crumbled feta, or chopped fresh herbs.

This avocado toast on whole grain bread is suitable for a fatty liver diet for seniors for the following reasons:

• Whole grain bread provides complex carbohydrates, fiber, and B vitamins.
• Avocado is a healthy source of monounsaturated fats, which can help reduce inflammation and support liver health.
• The olive oil and lemon juice add additional healthy fats and antioxidants.
• The optional toppings, such as tomatoes, radishes, and herbs, provide additional vitamins, minerals, and fiber.
• The dish is low in sodium and can be easily adjusted to meet individual dietary needs.

This simple and nutritious breakfast or snack can be a great option for seniors with fatty liver disease. The combination of healthy fats, fiber, and complex carbohydrates can help promote feelings of fullness and support overall liver function.

As always, it's best to consult with a healthcare professional for personalized dietary recommendations.

15. Smoothie with spinach, banana, and almond milk

Ingredients:

- 1 cup unsweetened almond milk
- 1 cup fresh spinach leaves
- 1 ripe banana, frozen
- 1 tbsp ground flaxseed (optional)
- 1 tsp honey (optional)

Instructions:

1. In a high·speed blender, combine the almond milk, fresh spinach leaves, frozen banana, and ground flaxseed (if using).

2. Blend the ingredients on high speed until the mixture is smooth and creamy.

3. Taste the smoothie and add a teaspoon of honey if desired, to provide a slight sweetness.

4. Pour the smoothie into a glass and enjoy immediately.

This spinach, banana, and almond milk smoothie is suitable for a fatty liver diet for seniors for the following reasons:

- Spinach is a nutrient·dense leafy green that is high in vitamins, minerals, and antioxidants, which can support liver health.
- Bananas are a good source of potassium, fiber, and natural sweetness.
- Almond milk is a dairy·free, low·calorie alternative to regular milk that is low in saturated fat.
- The optional ground flaxseed provides a source of healthy omega·3 fatty acids.
- The optional honey provides a natural sweetener, which can help satisfy a sweet craving without added sugars.
- The smoothie is low in sodium and can be easily adjusted to meet individual dietary needs.

This smoothie can be a refreshing and nutritious breakfast or snack option for seniors with fatty liver disease. The combination of leafy greens, fruit, and healthy fats can help support overall liver function and general health.

As always, it's best to consult with a healthcare professional for personalized dietary recommendations.

16. Roasted Brussels sprouts

Ingredients:

• 1 lb Brussels sprouts, trimmed and halved
• 2 tbsp olive oil
• 1 tsp garlic powder
• 1/2 tsp salt
• 1/4 tsp black pepper

Instructions:

1. Preheat the oven to 400°F.

2. In a large bowl, toss the trimmed and halved Brussels sprouts with the olive oil, garlic powder, salt, and black pepper until the sprouts are evenly coated.

3. Spread the seasoned Brussels sprouts in a single layer on a baking sheet.

4. Roast the Brussels sprouts in the preheated oven for 20•25 minutes, tossing halfway, until they are tender and lightly browned.

5. Serve the roasted Brussels sprouts hot.

This roasted Brussels sprouts dish is suitable for a fatty liver diet for seniors for the following reasons:

• Brussels sprouts are a cruciferous vegetable that is high in fiber, vitamins, and antioxidants, which can support liver health.
• The dish is roasted, which is a healthier cooking method compared to frying.
• The use of olive oil provides a healthy source of monounsaturated fats.
• The seasoning with garlic powder, salt, and pepper adds flavor without the need for excessive sodium.
• Brussels sprouts are low in calories and can be easily incorporated into a balanced diet.

Roasted Brussels sprouts can be a delicious and nutritious side dish or addition to a meal for seniors with fatty liver disease. The fiber, vitamins, and antioxidants in the Brussels sprouts can help support overall liver function.

As always, it's best to consult with a healthcare professional for personalized dietary recommendations.

17. Sautéed kale with garlic

Ingredients:

• 1 lb kale, stems removed and leaves chopped
• 1 tbsp olive oil
• 3 cloves garlic, minced
• 1/4 tsp red pepper flakes (optional)
• Salt and pepper to taste

Instructions:

1. In a large skillet or wok, heat the olive oil over medium heat.

2. Add the minced garlic to the skillet and sauté for 1•2 minutes, until fragrant.

3. Add the chopped kale leaves to the skillet. Sauté the kale, stirring frequently, for 5•7 minutes, until it is wilted and tender.

4. If using, sprinkle the red pepper flakes over the sautéed kale.

5. Season the kale with salt and pepper to taste.

6. Serve the sautéed kale warm.

This sautéed kale with garlic dish is suitable for a fatty liver diet for seniors for the following reasons:

• Kale is a nutrient•dense leafy green that is high in fiber, vitamins, and antioxidants, which can support liver health.
• The dish is sautéed, which is a healthy cooking method that preserves the nutrients in the kale.
• The use of olive oil provides a healthy source of monounsaturated fats.
• The garlic adds flavor without the need for excessive sodium.
• The optional red pepper flakes can provide a slight kick of heat without significantly increasing sodium.
• The meal is low in calories and can be easily incorporated into a balanced diet.

Sautéed kale with garlic can be a delicious and nutritious side dish or addition to a meal for seniors with fatty liver disease. The fiber, vitamins, and antioxidants in the kale can help support overall liver function.

18. Baked sweet potato fries

Ingredients:

• 2 medium sweet potatoes, peeled and cut into 1/2•inch thick fries
• 1 tbsp olive oil
• 1 tsp paprika
• 1/2 tsp garlic powder
• 1/4 tsp salt
• 1/4 tsp black pepper

Instructions:

1. Preheat the oven to 400°F.

2. In a large bowl, toss the sweet potato fries with the olive oil, paprika, garlic powder, salt, and black pepper until the fries are evenly coated.

3. Spread the seasoned sweet potato fries in a single layer on a baking sheet lined with parchment paper.

4. Bake the fries in the preheated oven for 20•25 minutes, flipping them halfway, until they are tender and lightly browned. Serve the baked sweet potato fries hot.

This baked sweet potato fries recipe is suitable for a fatty liver diet for seniors for the following reasons:

• Sweet potatoes are a nutrient•dense carbohydrate source that is high in fiber, vitamins, and antioxidants, which can support liver health.

• The dish is baked, which is a healthier cooking method compared to frying.

• The use of olive oil provides a healthy source of monounsaturated fats.

• The seasoning with paprika, garlic powder, salt, and pepper adds flavor without the need for excessive sodium.

• Sweet potato fries are a lower•calorie alternative to traditional French fries.

Baked sweet potato fries can be a delicious and nutritious side dish or snack for seniors with fatty liver disease. The fiber, vitamins, and antioxidants in the sweet potatoes can help support overall liver function.

19. Quinoa or brown rice pilaf

Ingredients:

- 1 cup uncooked quinoa or brown rice
- 2 cups low•sodium vegetable or chicken broth
- 1 tbsp olive oil
- 1 onion, diced
- 2 cloves garlic, minced
- 1 cup diced vegetables (such as carrots, bell peppers, or zucchini)
- 1/4 cup chopped fresh parsley
- 1 tsp dried thyme
- Salt and pepper to taste

Instructions:

1. In a medium saucepan, combine the quinoa or brown rice and broth. Bring to a boil, then reduce heat, cover, and simmer for 15•20 minutes, until the grains are tender and the liquid is absorbed.

2. In a separate skillet, heat the olive oil over medium heat. Add the diced onion and sauté for 3•4 minutes, until translucent.

3. Add the minced garlic and diced vegetables to the skillet. Sauté for an additional 5•7 minutes, until the vegetables are tender.

4. Fluff the cooked quinoa or brown rice with a fork and transfer it to the skillet with the sautéed vegetables.

5. Stir in the chopped parsley and dried thyme. Season with salt and pepper to taste. Serve the quinoa or brown rice pilaf warm.

This quinoa or brown rice pilaf is suitable for a fatty liver diet for seniors for the following reasons:

- Quinoa and brown rice are whole grains that are high in fiber, complex carbohydrates, and B vitamins, which can support liver health.
- The variety of vegetables, such as carrots, bell peppers, and zucchini, provide a range of vitamins, minerals, and antioxidants.
- The use of olive oil provides a healthy source of monounsaturated fats.
- The dish is low in sodium, as it uses low•sodium broth and minimal added salt.
- The meal is low in calories and can be easily adjusted to meet individual dietary needs.

This flavorful and nutritious pilaf can be a great option for seniors with fatty liver disease. It can be served as a main dish or a side to complement other lean protein sources

20. Steamed or roasted vegetables (broccoli, cauliflower, carrots, etc.)

Ingredients:

• 1 head broccoli, cut into florets
• 1 head cauliflower, cut into florets
• 3 carrots, peeled and sliced
• 1 tbsp olive oil (for roasting)
• Salt and pepper to taste

Instructions:

For Steamed Vegetables:

1. Fill a large pot with 1•2 inches of water and bring to a boil.
2. Place the broccoli, cauliflower, and carrot slices in a steamer basket and lower it into the pot.
3. Cover and steam the vegetables for 5•7 minutes, until they are tender but still crisp.
4. Remove the steamed vegetables from the pot and season with salt and pepper to taste.

For Roasted Vegetables:

1. Preheat the oven to 400°F.
2. Toss the broccoli, cauliflower, and carrot slices with the olive oil in a large bowl. Season with salt and pepper.
3. Spread the vegetables in a single layer on a baking sheet.
4. Roast the vegetables for 20•25 minutes, tossing halfway, until they are tender and lightly browned.

These steamed or roasted vegetables are suitable for a fatty liver diet for seniors for the following reasons:

• Broccoli, cauliflower, and carrots are nutrient•dense vegetables that are high in fiber, vitamins, and antioxidants, which can support liver health.
• The steaming or roasting cooking methods preserve the nutrients in the vegetables without the need for added fats or oils.
• The use of olive oil in the roasted version provides a healthy source of monounsaturated fats.
• The dish is low in sodium, as it only requires a minimal amount of salt for seasoning.
• The vegetables are low in calories and can be easily incorporated into a balanced diet.

These simple and versatile vegetable dishes can be a great option for seniors with fatty liver disease. They can be served as a side or incorporated into other meals.

21. Fresh fruit salad

Ingredients:

• 1 cup diced pineapple
• 1 cup diced mango
• 1 cup diced strawberries
• 1 cup blueberries
• 1 cup diced kiwi
• 1 tbsp fresh lemon juice
• 1 tbsp honey (optional)

Instructions:

1. In a large bowl, combine the diced pineapple, mango, strawberries, blueberries, and kiwi.

2. Drizzle the fresh lemon juice over the fruit and gently toss to coat.

3. If desired, drizzle the honey over the fruit salad and toss lightly to combine.

4. Serve the fresh fruit salad chilled or at room temperature.

This fresh fruit salad is suitable for a fatty liver diet for seniors for the following reasons:

• The variety of fruits, such as pineapple, mango, strawberries, blueberries, and kiwi, provide a wide range of vitamins, minerals, and antioxidants that can support liver health.

• The fruits are low in calories and high in fiber, which can help promote feelings of fullness and support overall health.

• The lemon juice adds a refreshing, tart flavor without the need for added sugars.

• The optional honey provides a natural sweetener, which can help satisfy a sweet craving without excessive added sugars.

• The dish is low in sodium and can be easily adjusted to meet individual dietary needs.

This colorful and nutritious fruit salad can be a great option for seniors with fatty liver disease. It can be enjoyed as a refreshing snack or a light dessert.

22. Mixed nuts and seeds

Ingredients:

1. Healthy Fats: Nuts and seeds are rich in healthy unsaturated fats, such as monounsaturated and polyunsaturated fats. These healthy fats can help reduce inflammation and support liver health.

2. Protein: Nuts and seeds provide a good source of plant•based protein, which can help maintain muscle mass and support overall health.

3. Fiber: Many nuts and seeds are high in fiber, which can help promote feelings of fullness and support digestive health.

4. Antioxidants: Nuts and seeds contain a variety of antioxidants, such as vitamin E, that can help protect the liver from oxidative stress.

Some recommended nuts and seeds for a fatty liver diet include:

• Walnuts
• Almonds
• Pecans
• Pistachios
• Pumpkin seeds
• Chia seeds
• Flaxseeds

When incorporating mixed nuts and seeds into a fatty liver diet for seniors, it's important to watch portion sizes, as they are calorie•dense. A serving size is typically 1/4 cup of nuts or 2 tablespoons of seeds.

It's also best to choose unsalted or low•sodium varieties to limit sodium intake. Seniors with fatty liver disease should consult with a healthcare professional for personalized dietary recommendations.

Overall, mixed nuts and seeds can be a nutritious and satisfying snack option that can support liver health and overall well•being for seniors with fatty liver disease.

23. Hummus with veggie sticks

Ingredients:

- 1 (15 oz) can chickpeas, drained and rinsed
- 2 tbsp tahini (sesame seed paste)
- 2 tbsp fresh lemon juice
- 1 garlic clove, minced
- 2 tbsp olive oil
- 1/4 tsp ground cumin
- Salt and pepper to taste
- Assorted raw vegetable sticks (such as carrots, celery, cucumber, bell peppers)

Instructions:

1. In a food processor or high•powered blender, combine the drained and rinsed chickpeas, tahini, lemon juice, garlic, olive oil, and cumin. Blend until smooth and creamy.

2. Season the hummus with salt and pepper to taste.

3. Transfer the hummus to a serving bowl.

4. Arrange the assorted raw vegetable sticks around the bowl of hummus.

This hummus with veggie sticks is suitable for a fatty liver diet for seniors for the following reasons:

- Chickpeas, the main ingredient in hummus, are a good source of plant•based protein, fiber, and complex carbohydrates, which can support liver health.

- Tahini provides healthy unsaturated fats from sesame seeds.

- The lemon juice and garlic add flavor without the need for excessive sodium.

- The raw vegetable sticks, such as carrots, celery, cucumber, and bell peppers, are low in calories and high in fiber, vitamins, and antioxidants.

- The dish is low in sodium and can be easily adjusted to meet individual dietary needs.

This nutritious and satisfying snack can be a great option for seniors with fatty liver disease. The combination of protein, fiber, and healthy fats from the hummus, paired with the nutrient•dense vegetables, can help promote feelings of fullness and support overall liver function.

24. Greek yogurt with granola

Ingredients:

• 1 cup plain Greek yogurt
• 1/2 cup low•sugar granola
• 1/2 cup fresh berries (such as blueberries, raspberries, or strawberries)
• 1 tsp honey (optional)

Instructions:

1. In a serving bowl, place the plain Greek yogurt.

2. Top the yogurt with the low•sugar granola.

3. Scatter the fresh berries over the granola.

4. If desired, drizzle a small amount of honey over the top.

This Greek yogurt with granola dish is suitable for a fatty liver diet for seniors for the following reasons:

• Greek yogurt is a high•protein, low•fat dairy product that can help support liver health.

• Low•sugar granola provides complex carbohydrates, fiber, and a crunchy texture without excessive added sugars.

• Fresh berries are low in calories and high in fiber, vitamins, and antioxidants.

• The optional honey provides a natural sweetener, which can help satisfy a sweet craving without added sugars.

• The dish is low in sodium and can be easily adjusted to meet individual dietary needs.

This simple and nutritious breakfast or snack can be a great option for seniors with fatty liver disease. The combination of protein, fiber, and healthy carbohydrates can help promote feelings of fullness and support overall liver function.

When selecting a granola, it's important to choose a low•sugar variety, as many commercial granolas can be high in added sugars. Alternatively, you can make your own homemade granola with minimal added sweeteners.

25. Hard•boiled eggs

Ingredients:

• Large eggs

Instructions:
1. Place the eggs in a single layer in a saucepan and cover with cold water by 1 inch.

2. Bring the water to a boil over high heat.

3. Once the water reaches a full boil, remove the pan from the heat and cover. Let the eggs sit in the hot water for 12 minutes.

4. Drain the hot water and cover the eggs with cold water to stop the cooking.

5. Let the eggs sit in the cold water for 5 minutes before peeling.

Tips:
• Hard•boiled eggs are a great source of protein that is easy to digest, which is important for those with fatty liver disease.

• The yolks contain healthy fats and nutrients like choline that can help support liver health.

• Avoid adding salt, as sodium should be limited on a fatty liver diet.

• Enjoy the hard•boiled eggs on their own or use them in salads, as a snack, or as part of a balanced meal.

26. Grilled tuna with roasted bell peppers

Ingredients:

• 4 (4•6 oz) tuna steaks
• 2 bell peppers (any color), sliced into strips
• 1 tbsp olive oil
• 1 tsp dried oregano
• 1/2 tsp garlic powder
• Salt and pepper to taste

Instructions:

1. Preheat grill or grill pan to medium•high heat.

2. In a baking dish, toss the bell pepper strips with the olive oil, oregano, garlic powder, salt, and pepper.

3. Roast the bell peppers in the oven at 400°F for 15•20 minutes, stirring halfway, until softened and lightly charred.

4. Season the tuna steaks with a bit of salt and pepper.

5. Grill the tuna for 3•4 minutes per side, or until it reaches your desired doneness. Be careful not to overcook.

6. Serve the grilled tuna immediately, topped with the roasted bell peppers.

Tips:

• Tuna is an excellent source of lean protein and omega•3 fatty acids, which are beneficial for liver health.

• Bell peppers are rich in antioxidants and can help reduce inflammation.

• This dish is low in sodium and carbs, making it a great option for a fatty liver diet.

• Pair it with a side of steamed vegetables or a simple salad for a complete, liver•friendly meal.

27. Vegetable and bean chili

Ingredients:

• 1 tbsp olive oil
• 1 onion, diced
• 3 cloves garlic, minced
• 1 red bell pepper, diced
• 1 zucchini, diced
• 1 can (15 oz) black beans, rinsed and drained
• 1 can (15 oz) kidney beans, rinsed and drained
• 1 can (28 oz) diced tomatoes
• 2 tbsp chili powder
• 1 tsp ground cumin
• 1 tsp dried oregano
• 1/4 tsp cayenne pepper (optional, for spice)
• Salt and pepper to taste

Instructions:

1. In a large pot or Dutch oven, heat the olive oil over medium heat. Add the onion and sauté for 5 minutes until translucent.

2. Add the garlic, bell pepper, and zucchini. Sauté for another 5 minutes, stirring occasionally.

3. Stir in the black beans, kidney beans, diced tomatoes, chili powder, cumin, oregano, and cayenne (if using). Season with salt and pepper to taste.

4. Bring the chili to a simmer and let it cook for 20•25 minutes, stirring occasionally, until the vegetables are tender and the flavors have melded.

5. Serve the chili hot, garnished with fresh cilantro or green onions if desired.

Tips:
• Beans are an excellent source of fiber and plant•based protein, which are important for a fatty liver diet.
• Vegetables like bell peppers and zucchini provide antioxidants and nutrients to support liver health.
• This chili is low in sodium and can be easily adjusted to suit individual dietary needs.
• Serve with a side of whole grain crackers or a small portion of brown rice for a complete, balanced meal.

28. Quinoa and black bean salad

Ingredients:

• 1 cup uncooked quinoa, rinsed
• 1 can (15 oz) black beans, rinsed and drained
• 1 cup diced cucumber
• 1 cup diced tomatoes
• 1/2 cup diced red onion
• 1/4 cup chopped fresh cilantro
• 2 tbsp olive oil
• 2 tbsp lime juice
• 1 tsp ground cumin
• 1/4 tsp cayenne pepper (optional, for spice)
• Salt and pepper to taste

Instructions:

1. Cook the quinoa according to package instructions. Allow to cool completely.

2. In a large bowl, combine the cooked quinoa, black beans, cucumber, tomatoes, red onion, and cilantro.

3. In a small bowl, whisk together the olive oil, lime juice, cumin, and cayenne (if using). Season with salt and pepper.

4. Pour the dressing over the quinoa and bean mixture and toss gently to coat.

5. Refrigerate the salad for at least 30 minutes to allow the flavors to meld.

6. Serve chilled or at room temperature.

Tips:
• Quinoa is a gluten•free, high•protein grain that is easy to digest, making it a great choice for a fatty liver diet.
• Black beans are a good source of fiber and plant•based protein, which can help support liver health.
• The vegetables provide antioxidants and nutrients that can help reduce inflammation.
• The lime juice and olive oil in the dressing provide healthy fats that are beneficial for the liver.
• This salad can be made ahead of time and keeps well in the refrigerator for up to 4 days.

29. Turkey lettuce wraps

Ingredients:

- 1 lb ground turkey
- 1 tbsp olive oil
- 1 onion, diced
- 3 cloves garlic, minced
- 1 tbsp low•sodium soy sauce or tamari
- 1 tsp ground ginger
- 1/2 tsp red pepper flakes (optional, for spice)
- Salt and pepper to taste
- 1 head of romaine or butter lettuce, leaves separated

For the Sauce:
- 2 tbsp tahini
- 2 tbsp rice vinegar
- 1 tbsp honey
- 1 tbsp water
- 1 tsp sesame oil
- Salt and pepper to taste

Instructions:

1. In a large skillet, heat the olive oil over medium•high heat. Add the ground turkey and cook, breaking it up with a wooden spoon, until browned, about 5•7 minutes.

2. Add the onion and garlic to the skillet and cook for another 2•3 minutes until the onion is translucent.

3. Stir in the soy sauce, ginger, and red pepper flakes (if using). Season with salt and pepper to taste. In a small bowl, whisk together all the sauce ingredients until well combined.

5. To assemble the wraps, place a few spoonfuls of the turkey mixture into a lettuce leaf. Drizzle with the tahini sauce. Fold the lettuce leaf around the filling and enjoy.

Tips:
- Ground turkey is a lean protein that is easy to digest, making it a great choice for a fatty liver diet.
- Lettuce leaves provide a low•carb, high•fiber wrap option.
- The tahini•based sauce adds healthy fats and a creamy texture to the wraps.
- This recipe is low in sodium and can be easily adjusted to suit individual dietary needs.
- Serve the wraps with a side of steamed vegetables or a simple salad for a complete, liver•friendly meal.

30. Baked potato with steamed broccoli and salsa

Ingredients:

• 4 medium russet potatoes
• 1 head of broccoli, cut into florets
• 1 cup salsa (look for low•sodium options)
• 2 tbsp plain Greek yogurt (optional)
• Salt and pepper to taste

Instructions:

1. Preheat the oven to 400°F.

2. Wash the potatoes and prick them several times with a fork. Place the potatoes directly on the oven rack and bake for 50•60 minutes, or until a knife can easily pierce through the center.

3. While the potatoes are baking, steam the broccoli florets in a steamer basket or in the microwave until tender, about 5•7 minutes.

4. Once the potatoes are cooked, remove them from the oven and let them cool for a few minutes.

5. Slice the potatoes open and top with the steamed broccoli, salsa, and a dollop of Greek yogurt (if using). Season with salt and pepper to taste.

Tips:

• Baked potatoes are a great source of complex carbohydrates and fiber, which can help support a healthy liver.

• Broccoli is rich in antioxidants and can help reduce inflammation in the body.

• Salsa provides a flavorful, low•calorie topping that is also low in sodium.

• The Greek yogurt adds a creamy texture and a boost of protein.

• This dish is easy to prepare and can be customized to individual dietary needs.

31. Grilled chicken with roasted butternut squash

Ingredients:

• 4 boneless, skinless chicken breasts
• 1 medium butternut squash, peeled, seeded, and cubed
• 2 tbsp olive oil, divided
• 1 tsp dried thyme
• 1 tsp garlic powder
• Salt and pepper to taste

Instructions:

1. Preheat the oven to 400°F.

2. In a large bowl, toss the cubed butternut squash with 1 tbsp of the olive oil, thyme, garlic powder, salt, and pepper.

3. Spread the seasoned squash cubes on a baking sheet and roast for 25•30 minutes, or until tender and lightly browned, stirring halfway.

4. While the squash is roasting, brush the chicken breasts with the remaining 1 tbsp of olive oil and season with salt and pepper.

5. Grill the chicken over medium•high heat for 5•7 minutes per side, or until the internal temperature reaches 165°F.

6. Serve the grilled chicken alongside the roasted butternut squash.

Tips:
• Chicken is a lean protein that is easy to digest, making it a great choice for a fatty liver diet.
• Butternut squash is rich in fiber, vitamins, and antioxidants that can support liver health.
• The combination of grilled chicken and roasted squash provides a balanced, nutrient•dense meal.
• This dish is low in sodium and can be easily adjusted to suit individual dietary needs.
• Consider adding a side of steamed greens or a simple salad for an even more well•rounded meal.

32. Baked tilapia with lemon and dill

Ingredients:

• 4 tilapia fillets (about 4•6 oz each)
• 2 tbsp olive oil
• 2 tbsp freshly squeezed lemon juice
• 2 tsp dried dill
• 1 tsp garlic powder
• Salt and pepper to taste
• Lemon wedges for serving

Instructions:

1. Preheat the oven to 400°F.

2. Place the tilapia fillets in a baking dish or on a parchment•lined baking sheet.

3. In a small bowl, whisk together the olive oil, lemon juice, dill, and garlic powder. Season with salt and pepper.

4. Drizzle the lemon•dill mixture over the tilapia fillets, making sure to evenly coat the fish.

5. Bake the tilapia for 15•18 minutes, or until the fish flakes easily with a fork and is opaque throughout.

6. Serve the baked tilapia immediately, garnished with fresh lemon wedges.

Tips:
• Tilapia is a lean, mild•flavored fish that is a great source of protein and omega•3 fatty acids, both of which are beneficial for liver health.

• Lemon and dill provide a bright, flavorful seasoning without the need for added salt or heavy sauces.

• This dish is low in calories and carbs, making it a suitable option for a fatty liver diet.

• Pair the baked tilapia with roasted vegetables or a simple salad for a complete, liver•friendly meal.

• Leftovers can be stored in the refrigerator for up to 3 days and reheated gently before serving.

33. Vegetable fried rice with tofu

Ingredients:

- 1 block (14 oz) firm or extra-firm tofu, diced
- 2 tbsp low-sodium soy sauce or tamari
- 1 tbsp sesame oil
- 2 tbsp olive oil, divided
- 1 cup diced carrots
- 1 cup diced bell peppers
- 1 cup diced mushrooms
- 1 cup frozen peas
- 3 cloves garlic, minced
- 1 tsp grated ginger
- 3 cups cooked brown rice, cooled
- 2 eggs, lightly beaten
- 2 tbsp chopped green onions
- Salt and pepper to taste

Instructions:

1. In a small bowl, toss the diced tofu with the soy sauce and sesame oil. Set aside.

2. Heat 1 tbsp of the olive oil in a large skillet or wok over medium-high heat. Add the tofu and cook, stirring occasionally, until lightly browned on all sides, about 5-7 minutes. Transfer the tofu to a plate and set aside.

3. Add the remaining 1 tbsp of olive oil to the skillet. Add the carrots, bell peppers, mushrooms, and peas. Sauté for 5-7 minutes, until the vegetables are tender.

4. Push the vegetables to the side of the skillet and pour the beaten eggs into the empty space. Scramble the eggs, then mix them into the vegetables.

5. Add the garlic and ginger to the skillet and cook for 1 minute, until fragrant.

6. Add the cooked brown rice and the sautéed tofu to the skillet. Toss everything together until well combined and heated through.

7. Remove from heat and stir in the chopped green onions. Season with salt and pepper to taste. Serve the vegetable fried rice with tofu immediately.

Tips:
- Tofu is a great source of plant-based protein that is easy to digest, making it a good choice for a fatty liver diet.

- The vegetables provide fiber, vitamins, and antioxidants that can support liver health.

- Brown rice is a whole grain that is higher in fiber and nutrients compared to white rice.

- This dish is low in sodium and can be easily adjusted to suit individual dietary needs.

34. Lentil and vegetable soup

Ingredients:

• 1 tbsp olive oil
• 1 onion, diced
• 3 cloves garlic, minced
• 2 carrots, peeled and diced
• 2 celery stalks, diced
• 1 cup green or brown lentils, rinsed
• 6 cups low•sodium vegetable broth
• 1 (14.5 oz) can diced tomatoes
• 2 cups chopped kale or spinach
• 1 tsp dried thyme
• 1 tsp dried oregano
• Salt and pepper to taste

Instructions:

1. In a large pot or Dutch oven, heat the olive oil over medium heat. Add the onion and sauté for 5 minutes until translucent.

2. Add the garlic, carrots, and celery. Sauté for another 3•4 minutes.

3. Stir in the lentils, vegetable broth, diced tomatoes, kale/spinach, thyme, and oregano. Season with salt and pepper to taste.

4. Bring the soup to a boil, then reduce the heat and let it simmer for 25•30 minutes, or until the lentils are tender.

5. Taste and adjust seasoning as needed. Serve the lentil and vegetable soup hot, garnished with additional chopped kale/spinach or a sprinkle of parmesan cheese (if desired).

Tips:
• Lentils are an excellent source of plant•based protein and fiber, both of which are important for a fatty liver diet.
• The vegetables, such as carrots, celery, and greens, provide antioxidants and nutrients that can support liver health.
• This soup is low in sodium and can be easily adjusted to suit individual dietary needs.
• For added protein, you can also stir in some cooked chicken or turkey towards the end of the cooking time.
• Serve the soup with a side of whole grain crackers or a small portion of whole grain bread for a complete, balanced meal.

35. Whole wheat pita with hummus and vegetables

Ingredients:

• 4 whole wheat pita breads
• 1 cup hummus (look for low•sodium options)
• 1 cup sliced cucumber
• 1 cup sliced bell peppers
• 1 cup shredded carrots
• 1/2 cup sliced radishes
• 2 tbsp chopped fresh parsley or cilantro (optional)

Instructions:
1. Toast the whole wheat pita breads until lightly golden and crisp.

2. Spread about 1/4 cup of hummus onto each pita bread.

3. Top the hummus•covered pitas with the sliced cucumber, bell peppers, shredded carrots, and sliced radishes.

4. Sprinkle the chopped parsley or cilantro over the top, if desired.

5. Serve the pita sandwiches immediately.

Tips:
• Whole wheat pita provides complex carbohydrates and fiber, which are important for a fatty liver diet.

• Hummus is a great source of plant•based protein and healthy fats from the tahini and olive oil.

• The fresh vegetables add a crunchy texture and provide antioxidants, vitamins, and minerals that can support liver health.

• This recipe is low in sodium and can be easily customized to individual preferences.

• For added protein, you can also include a few slices of grilled chicken or turkey breast.

• Serve the pita sandwiches with a side of fresh fruit or a small salad for a complete, balanced meal.

36. Overnight oats with berries and chia seeds

Ingredients:

• 1 cup old•fashioned rolled oats
• 1 cup unsweetened almond milk (or milk of your choice)
• 2 tbsp chia seeds
• 1 tbsp honey (optional)
• 1 cup mixed berries (such as blueberries, raspberries, and/or blackberries)

Instructions:

1. In a medium•sized bowl or mason jar, combine the rolled oats, almond milk, chia seeds, and honey (if using). Stir well to combine.

2. Cover the bowl or seal the mason jar and refrigerate overnight, or for at least 4 hours.

3. In the morning, give the overnight oats a stir. Top with the mixed berries.

4. Serve chilled or at room temperature.

Tips:
• Oats are a whole grain that are high in fiber, which can help support liver health.

• Chia seeds are a great source of omega•3 fatty acids, which can also benefit the liver.

• Berries are packed with antioxidants and vitamins that can help reduce inflammation.

• The honey (if using) provides a natural sweetener, but you can also omit it or use a small amount of maple syrup or stevia instead.

• This recipe is low in sodium and can be easily adjusted to suit individual dietary needs.

• For added protein, you can stir in a scoop of plain Greek yogurt or a tablespoon of almond butter.

• Prepare the overnight oats in advance for a quick and nutritious breakfast option.

37. Veggie omelet with tomatoes and spinach

Ingredients:

- 3 large eggs
- 2 tbsp unsweetened almond milk (or milk of your choice)
- 1 tsp olive oil
- 1/2 cup diced tomatoes
- 1 cup fresh spinach, chopped
- 1 tbsp grated parmesan cheese (optional)
- Salt and pepper to taste

Instructions:

1. In a small bowl, whisk together the eggs and almond milk. Season with a pinch of salt and pepper.

2. Heat the olive oil in a nonstick skillet over medium heat.

3. Pour the egg mixture into the skillet and let it cook for 2•3 minutes, or until the edges start to set.

4. Gently lift the edges of the omelet with a spatula and tilt the pan to allow the uncooked egg to flow to the edges.

5. Once the bottom is set but the top is still slightly runny, add the diced tomatoes and chopped spinach to one half of the omelet.

6. Fold the other half of the omelet over the vegetable•filled half. Cook for an additional 1•2 minutes, or until the omelet is set. Carefully slide the omelet onto a plate and top with the grated parmesan cheese, if using.

Tips:
- Eggs are a great source of protein that is easy to digest, making them a good choice for a fatty liver diet.
- Tomatoes and spinach provide antioxidants, vitamins, and minerals that can support liver health.
- The parmesan cheese adds a boost of flavor and a small amount of healthy fat.
- This omelet is low in sodium and can be easily customized with other vegetables, such as bell peppers or mushrooms.
- Serve the omelet with a side of whole grain toast or a small salad for a complete, balanced meal.

38. Cottage cheese with fresh fruits

Ingredients:

• 1 cup low•fat or non•fat cottage cheese
• 1 cup mixed fresh fruits (such as berries, diced apple, diced pear, or melon)
• 1 tsp honey (optional)
• Cinnamon (optional)

Instructions:

1. In a bowl, scoop out the cottage cheese.

2. Top the cottage cheese with the mixed fresh fruits.

3. If desired, drizzle the honey over the top and sprinkle with a dash of cinnamon.

4. Serve immediately.

Tips:
• Cottage cheese is a great source of protein that is easy to digest, making it a good choice for a fatty liver diet.

• Fresh fruits provide a variety of vitamins, minerals, and antioxidants that can support liver health.

• The honey (if using) adds a touch of natural sweetness, but you can also omit it or use a small amount of maple syrup or stevia instead.

• Cinnamon is an optional addition that can provide a warm, comforting flavor.

• This dish is low in sodium and can be easily customized with your choice of seasonal fruits.

• For added fiber and healthy fats, you can also sprinkle a tablespoon of chopped nuts or seeds over the top.

• Enjoy this cottage cheese and fruit combination as a snack or a light, nutritious breakfast.

39. Whole wheat toast with avocado and tomato

Ingredients:

• 2 slices of whole wheat bread
• 1 ripe avocado, mashed
• 1 medium tomato, diced
• 1 tbsp fresh lemon juice
• 1 tsp olive oil
• Salt and pepper to taste

Instructions:

1. Toast the whole wheat bread until lightly golden.

2. In a small bowl, mash the avocado with the lemon juice, olive oil, and a pinch of salt and pepper.

3. Spread the mashed avocado evenly over the toasted whole wheat bread.

4. Top the avocado toast with the diced tomatoes.

5. Season the dish with additional salt and pepper to taste.

Tips:
• Whole wheat bread provides complex carbohydrates and fiber, which are important for a fatty liver diet.

• Avocado is a great source of healthy monounsaturated fats that can help support liver health.

• Tomatoes are rich in antioxidants, such as lycopene, that can also benefit the liver.

• The lemon juice and olive oil add flavor and healthy fats to the dish.

• This recipe is low in sodium and can be easily adjusted to suit individual dietary needs.

• For added protein, you can also top the avocado toast with a poached or hard•boiled egg.

• Serve the avocado and tomato toast as a light breakfast, snack, or part of a larger liver•friendly meal.

40. Green smoothie with spinach, pineapple, and almond milk

Ingredients:

• 1 cup unsweetened almond milk
• 1 cup fresh spinach leaves
• 1 cup frozen pineapple chunks
• 1 banana, frozen
• 1 tbsp ground flaxseed
• 1 tsp honey (optional)

Instructions:
1. In a high•speed blender, combine the almond milk, spinach, pineapple, banana, and flaxseed.

2. Blend on high speed until the mixture is smooth and creamy, about 1•2 minutes. If desired, add the honey and blend again briefly to incorporate. Pour the green smoothie into a glass and enjoy immediately.

Tips:
• Spinach is a nutrient•dense green that is rich in antioxidants and vitamins that can support liver health.

• Pineapple contains the enzyme bromelain, which can help reduce inflammation in the body.

• Almond milk is a dairy•free, low•calorie option that provides a creamy texture to the smoothie.

• Bananas add natural sweetness and creaminess, while the flaxseed provides a boost of omega•3 fatty acids.

• The honey (if using) provides a touch of natural sweetness, but you can also omit it or use a small amount of maple syrup or stevia instead.

• This smoothie is low in sodium and can be easily adjusted to suit individual dietary needs.

• For added protein, you can also include a scoop of plain Greek yogurt or a tablespoon of nut butter.

• Enjoy the green smoothie as a nutritious breakfast or snack.

41. Roasted cauliflower with garlic

Ingredients:

• 1 head of cauliflower, cut into florets
• 2 tbsp olive oil
• 3 cloves garlic, minced
• 1 tsp dried thyme
• 1/4 tsp cayenne pepper (optional, for a bit of heat)
• Salt and pepper to taste

Instructions:

1. Preheat the oven to 400°F.

2. In a large bowl, toss the cauliflower florets with the olive oil, minced garlic, dried thyme, and cayenne pepper (if using). Season with salt and pepper.

3. Spread the seasoned cauliflower in a single layer on a baking sheet lined with parchment paper.

4. Roast the cauliflower for 20•25 minutes, stirring halfway, until the florets are tender and lightly browned.

5. Serve the roasted cauliflower hot, garnished with additional fresh thyme or parsley, if desired.

Tips:
• Cauliflower is a cruciferous vegetable that is rich in antioxidants and fiber, both of which can support liver health.

• Garlic is a natural anti•inflammatory and can also provide benefits for the liver.

• The olive oil adds healthy monounsaturated fats to the dish.

• The optional cayenne pepper provides a subtle heat that can help stimulate digestion.

• This recipe is low in sodium and can be easily adjusted to suit individual dietary needs.

• Pair the roasted cauliflower with grilled or baked protein, such as chicken or fish, for a complete, liver•friendly meal.

• Leftovers can be stored in the refrigerator for up to 4 days and reheated gently before serving.

42. Sautéed Swiss chard with lemon

Ingredients:

• 1 bunch of Swiss chard, stems removed and leaves chopped
• 1 tbsp olive oil
• 2 cloves garlic, minced
• 1 tbsp freshly squeezed lemon juice
• Salt and pepper to taste

Instructions:
1. In a large skillet or sauté pan, heat the olive oil over medium heat.

2. Add the chopped Swiss chard leaves and sauté for 2•3 minutes, until they start to wilt.

3. Add the minced garlic and continue to sauté for another 1•2 minutes, until the garlic is fragrant.

4. Drizzle the lemon juice over the sautéed chard and toss to coat.

5. Season with salt and pepper to taste.

6. Serve the sautéed Swiss chard warm.

Tips:
• Swiss chard is a nutrient•dense leafy green that is rich in antioxidants, vitamins, and minerals that can support liver health.

• The lemon juice adds a bright, tangy flavor and provides a boost of vitamin C.

• This dish is low in sodium and can be easily adjusted to suit individual dietary needs.

• For added protein, you can top the sautéed chard with grilled chicken or salmon.

• Serve the chard as a side dish or incorporate it into a larger liver•friendly meal, such as a grain bowl or frittata.

• Leftovers can be stored in the refrigerator for up to 3 days and reheated gently before serving.

43. Baked zucchini fries

Ingredients:

• 2 medium zucchini, cut into 1/2•inch thick fry•shaped pieces
• 1 tbsp olive oil
• 1/2 cup grated parmesan cheese
• 1 tsp garlic powder
• 1 tsp dried oregano
• 1/4 tsp cayenne pepper (optional, for a bit of heat)
• Salt and pepper to taste

Instructions:
1. Preheat the oven to 400°F. Line a baking sheet with parchment paper.

2. In a large bowl, toss the zucchini fries with the olive oil until evenly coated.

3. In a shallow bowl, mix together the parmesan cheese, garlic powder, oregano, and cayenne pepper (if using).

4. Working in batches, dip the zucchini fries into the parmesan mixture, coating them evenly on all sides.

5. Arrange the coated zucchini fries in a single layer on the prepared baking sheet.

6. Bake for 18•22 minutes, flipping the fries halfway, until they are golden brown and crispy.

7. Remove the baked zucchini fries from the oven and season with salt and pepper to taste. Serve the zucchini fries hot, garnished with additional parmesan cheese or fresh herbs, if desired.

Tips:
• Zucchini is a low•calorie, high•fiber vegetable that can provide benefits for liver health.
• The parmesan cheese adds a savory, crispy coating without the need for heavy breading or frying.
• The garlic, oregano, and optional cayenne pepper provide flavor and a touch of heat.
• This recipe is low in sodium and can be easily adjusted to suit individual dietary needs.
• Pair the baked zucchini fries with grilled or baked protein, such as chicken or fish, for a complete, liver•friendly meal.
• Leftovers can be stored in the refrigerator for up to 3 days and reheated in the oven or air fryer to maintain their crispy texture.

44. Brown rice pilaf with vegetables

Ingredients:

• 1 cup uncooked brown rice
• 2 cups low•sodium vegetable or chicken broth
• 1 tbsp olive oil
• 1 onion, diced
• 2 carrots, peeled and diced
• 1 bell pepper, diced
• 1 cup sliced mushrooms
• 2 cloves garlic, minced
• 1 tsp dried thyme
• Salt and pepper to taste
• 2 tbsp chopped fresh parsley (optional)

Instructions:

1. In a medium saucepan, bring the brown rice and broth to a boil. Reduce heat, cover, and simmer for 25•30 minutes, or until the rice is tender and the liquid is absorbed. Fluff with a fork and set aside.

2. In a large skillet or sauté pan, heat the olive oil over medium heat. Add the onion and sauté for 3•4 minutes until translucent.

3. Add the carrots, bell pepper, mushrooms, and garlic. Sauté for an additional 5•7 minutes, until the vegetables are tender.

4. Stir the cooked brown rice into the vegetable mixture. Add the dried thyme and season with salt and pepper to taste.

5. Cook for 2•3 minutes, stirring occasionally, to allow the flavors to meld. Remove from heat and stir in the chopped fresh parsley, if using. Serve the brown rice pilaf warm.

Tips:
• Brown rice is a whole grain that is high in fiber, which can help support liver health.
• The variety of vegetables provides a range of antioxidants, vitamins, and minerals that can also benefit the liver.
• This dish is low in sodium and can be easily adjusted to suit individual dietary needs.
• For added protein, you can stir in some cooked chicken, shrimp, or tofu.
• Serve the brown rice pilaf as a main dish or as a side to grilled or baked fish or poultry.
• Leftovers can be stored in the refrigerator for up to 4 days and reheated gently before serving.

45. Roasted root vegetables (carrots, beets, parsnips)

Ingredients:

• 2 carrots, peeled and cut into 1•inch pieces
• 2 beets, peeled and cut into 1•inch pieces
• 2 parsnips, peeled and cut into 1•inch pieces
• 2 tbsp olive oil
• 1 tsp dried thyme
• 1 tsp garlic powder
• Salt and pepper to taste

Instructions:

1. Preheat the oven to 400°F. Line a large baking sheet with parchment paper.

2. In a large bowl, toss the prepared root vegetables (carrots, beets, and parsnips) with the olive oil, dried thyme, garlic powder, salt, and pepper until evenly coated.

3. Spread the seasoned root vegetables in a single layer on the prepared baking sheet.

4. Roast for 25•30 minutes, stirring halfway, until the vegetables are tender and lightly browned.

5. Remove the roasted root vegetables from the oven and serve hot.

Tips:
• Root vegetables like carrots, beets, and parsnips are rich in fiber, vitamins, and antioxidants that can support liver health.

• The olive oil provides healthy monounsaturated fats, while the thyme and garlic add flavor without the need for excessive sodium.

• This recipe is low in sodium and can be easily adjusted to suit individual dietary needs.

• For added protein, you can roast the root vegetables alongside chicken, salmon, or tofu.

• Serve the roasted root vegetables as a side dish or incorporate them into a larger liver•friendly meal, such as a grain bowl or salad.

• Leftovers can be stored in the refrigerator for up to 4 days and reheated in the oven or air fryer before serving.

46. Fresh fruit kebabs

Ingredients:

- 1 cup cubed pineapple
- 1 cup cubed watermelon
- 1 cup cubed cantaloupe
- 1 cup blueberries
- 1 cup strawberries, halved
- 1 tbsp honey (optional)

Instructions:
1. Wash and prepare the fruit. Cut the pineapple, watermelon, and cantaloupe into 1•inch cubes.

2. Thread the fruit onto skewers, alternating the different types of fruit.

3. If desired, drizzle the fruit kebabs with a small amount of honey.

4. Serve the fresh fruit kebabs chilled or at room temperature.

Tips:
- Fruit is an excellent source of vitamins, minerals, and antioxidants that can support liver health.

- The variety of fruits on the kebabs provides a range of nutrients and flavors.

- The honey (if using) adds a touch of natural sweetness, but you can also omit it or use a small amount of maple syrup or stevia instead.

- This recipe is low in sodium and can be easily adjusted to include your favorite seasonal fruits.

- Fruit kebabs make a refreshing and nutritious snack or dessert option for a fatty liver diet.

- Serve the fruit kebabs on their own or alongside a small portion of plain Greek yogurt or cottage cheese for added protein.

- Leftovers can be stored in the refrigerator for up to 3 days.

47. Trail mix with nuts, seeds, and dried fruits

Ingredients:

- 1/2 cup raw almonds
- 1/2 cup raw walnuts
- 1/4 cup raw pumpkin seeds
- 1/4 cup raw sunflower seeds
- 1/4 cup unsweetened dried cranberries
- 1/4 cup unsweetened dried apricots, chopped
- 1 tbsp unsweetened shredded coconut (optional)

Instructions:

1. In a large bowl, combine the almonds, walnuts, pumpkin seeds, sunflower seeds, dried cranberries, and dried apricots.

2. If using, stir in the unsweetened shredded coconut.

3. Mix all the ingredients together until well combined.

4. Transfer the trail mix to an airtight container or resealable bag for storage.

Tips:
- Nuts and seeds are excellent sources of healthy fats, protein, and fiber, which are all important for a fatty liver diet.

- Dried fruits provide natural sweetness and antioxidants, but be mindful of portion sizes as they are higher in sugar.

- The unsweetened coconut (if using) adds a nice texture and flavor without added sugar.

- This trail mix is low in sodium and can be easily customized to your taste preferences.

- Portion out the trail mix into individual servings for a convenient, on•the•go snack.

- Enjoy the trail mix on its own or sprinkle it over plain Greek yogurt or oatmeal for a nutritious breakfast or snack.

- Store the trail mix in an airtight container at room temperature for up to 2 weeks.

48. Cucumber and tomato salad with balsamic vinegar

Ingredients:

• 2 cups diced cucumber
• 1 cup diced tomatoes
• 1/4 cup thinly sliced red onion
• 2 tbsp balsamic vinegar
• 1 tbsp olive oil
• 1 tsp dried oregano
• Salt and pepper to taste

Instructions:
1. In a large bowl, combine the diced cucumber, tomatoes, and sliced red onion.

2. In a small bowl, whisk together the balsamic vinegar and olive oil.

3. Pour the balsamic vinaigrette over the cucumber and tomato mixture. Sprinkle with the dried oregano and season with salt and pepper to taste.

4. Gently toss the salad to coat the vegetables evenly with the dressing. Serve the cucumber and tomato salad chilled or at room temperature.

Tips:
• Cucumbers and tomatoes are both low•calorie, high•fiber vegetables that can provide benefits for liver health.

• The balsamic vinegar adds a tangy, flavorful dressing without the need for heavy oils or creams.

• The olive oil provides healthy monounsaturated fats to the salad.

• The dried oregano adds a touch of Mediterranean flavor.

• This salad is low in sodium and can be easily adjusted to suit individual dietary needs.

• For added protein, you can top the salad with grilled chicken, shrimp, or crumbled feta cheese.

• Serve the cucumber and tomato salad as a side dish or enjoy it on its own as a refreshing, liver•friendly snack. Leftovers can be stored in the refrigerator for up to 3 days.

49. Greek yogurt with fresh berries

Ingredients:

• 1 cup plain, low•fat or non•fat Greek yogurt
• 1 cup mixed fresh berries (such as blueberries, raspberries, and/or blackberries)
• 1 tsp honey (optional)
• 1 tbsp chopped walnuts or almonds (optional)

Instructions:
1. Scoop the Greek yogurt into a bowl or serving dish.

2. Top the yogurt with the mixed fresh berries.

3. If desired, drizzle the honey over the top of the berries and yogurt.

4. Sprinkle the chopped walnuts or almonds over the dish, if using.

5. Serve immediately.

Tips:
• Greek yogurt is a great source of protein that is easy to digest, making it a good choice for a fatty liver diet.

• Fresh berries are packed with antioxidants, vitamins, and fiber that can support liver health.

• The honey (if using) provides a touch of natural sweetness, but you can also omit it or use a small amount of maple syrup or stevia instead.

• The nuts add a crunchy texture and healthy fats to the dish.

• This recipe is low in sodium and can be easily adjusted to suit individual dietary needs.

• For added fiber, you can also stir in a tablespoon of ground flaxseed or chia seeds.

• Enjoy this Greek yogurt and berry parfait as a nutritious breakfast, snack, or dessert.

50. Deviled eggs

Ingredients:

• 6 hard•boiled eggs, peeled
• 2 tbsp plain, low•fat Greek yogurt
• 1 tsp Dijon mustard
• 1 tsp lemon juice
• 1/4 tsp paprika
• Salt and pepper to taste
• Chopped chives or parsley for garnish (optional)

Instructions:
1. Slice the hard•boiled eggs in half lengthwise and carefully remove the yolks, placing them in a small bowl.

2. In the bowl with the yolks, mash them with a fork. Add the Greek yogurt, Dijon mustard, lemon juice, paprika, and a pinch of salt and pepper. Mix well until the filling is smooth and creamy.

3. Spoon or pipe the yolk mixture back into the egg white halves.

4. Garnish the deviled eggs with chopped chives or parsley, if desired.

5. Refrigerate the deviled eggs until ready to serve.

Tips:
• Hard•boiled eggs are a great source of protein that is easy to digest, making them a good choice for a fatty liver diet.

• The Greek yogurt provides a creamy texture and a boost of protein without the need for high•fat mayonnaise.

• The Dijon mustard and lemon juice add flavor without added sodium.

• This recipe is low in sodium and can be easily adjusted to suit individual dietary needs.

• For added nutrition, you can also mix in a small amount of finely chopped spinach or bell peppers to the yolk mixture.

• Serve the deviled eggs as a snack or appetizer, or include them as part of a larger liver•friendly meal. Leftovers can be stored in the refrigerator for up to 3 days.

51. Grilled shrimp with roasted vegetables

Ingredients:

• 1 lb large shrimp, peeled and deveined
• 2 tbsp olive oil, divided
• 1 tsp garlic powder
• 1 tsp dried oregano
• Salt and pepper to taste
• 2 cups mixed vegetables (such as bell peppers, zucchini, and onions), cut into 1•inch pieces
• 1 lemon, cut into wedges for serving

Instructions:

1. Preheat the grill or grill pan to medium•high heat.

2. In a large bowl, toss the shrimp with 1 tbsp of the olive oil, garlic powder, dried oregano, and a pinch of salt and pepper.

3. In a separate bowl, toss the mixed vegetables with the remaining 1 tbsp of olive oil and season with salt and pepper.

4. Grill the shrimp for 2•3 minutes per side, or until they are opaque and cooked through.

5. Spread the seasoned vegetables on a baking sheet and roast in the oven at 400°F for 15•20 minutes, stirring halfway, until tender and lightly charred.

6. Serve the grilled shrimp and roasted vegetables immediately, with lemon wedges on the side.

Tips:
• Shrimp is a lean protein that is easy to digest, making it a great choice for a fatty liver diet.
• The variety of roasted vegetables provides a range of antioxidants, vitamins, and fiber that can support liver health.
• The olive oil adds healthy monounsaturated fats to the dish.
• This recipe is low in sodium and can be easily adjusted to suit individual dietary needs.
• For added flavor, you can also marinate the shrimp in a small amount of lemon juice or white wine before grilling.
• Serve the grilled shrimp and roasted vegetables over a bed of quinoa or brown rice for a complete, liver•friendly meal.
• Leftovers can be stored in the refrigerator for up to 3 days and reheated gently before serving.

52. Chickpea and vegetable soup

Ingredients:

- 1 tbsp olive oil
- 1 onion, diced
- 3 cloves garlic, minced
- 2 carrots, peeled and diced
- 2 celery stalks, diced
- 1 zucchini, diced
- 1 can (15 oz) chickpeas, rinsed and drained
- 4 cups low•sodium vegetable broth
- 1 tsp dried thyme
- 1 tsp dried oregano
- Salt and pepper to taste
- Chopped fresh parsley for garnish (optional)

Instructions:

1. In a large pot or Dutch oven, heat the olive oil over medium heat. Add the onion and sauté for 3•4 minutes until translucent.

2. Add the garlic, carrots, celery, and zucchini. Sauté for an additional 5 minutes, stirring occasionally.

3. Stir in the chickpeas, vegetable broth, thyme, and oregano. Season with salt and pepper to taste.

4. Bring the soup to a boil, then reduce the heat and let it simmer for 20•25 minutes, or until the vegetables are tender.

5. Ladle the chickpea and vegetable soup into bowls and garnish with chopped fresh parsley, if desired.

Tips:

• Chickpeas are an excellent source of plant•based protein and fiber, both of which are important for a fatty liver diet.

• The variety of vegetables provides antioxidants, vitamins, and minerals that can support liver health.

• The olive oil adds healthy monounsaturated fats to the soup.

• This recipe is low in sodium and can be easily adjusted to suit individual dietary needs.

• For added protein, you can also stir in some cooked chicken or turkey towards the end of the cooking time.

• Serve the chickpea and vegetable soup with a side of whole grain crackers or a small salad for a complete, liver•friendly meal.

• Leftovers can be stored in the refrigerator for up to 4 days and reheated gently before serving.

53. Quinoa tabbouleh salad

Ingredients:

• 1 cup uncooked quinoa, rinsed
• 1 cup chopped fresh parsley
• 1/2 cup chopped fresh mint
• 1 cup diced cucumber
• 1 cup diced tomatoes
• 1/4 cup diced red onion
• 2 tbsp olive oil
• 2 tbsp lemon juice
• 1 tsp ground cumin
• Salt and pepper to taste

Instructions:

1. Cook the quinoa according to package instructions. Allow to cool completely.

2. In a large bowl, combine the cooked quinoa, parsley, mint, cucumber, tomatoes, and red onion.

3. In a small bowl, whisk together the olive oil, lemon juice, cumin, salt, and pepper.

4. Pour the dressing over the quinoa mixture and toss gently to coat. Refrigerate for at least 30 minutes before serving to allow the flavors to meld.

This salad is a great option for a fatty liver diet for seniors for a few reasons:

• Quinoa is a whole grain that is high in fiber, protein, and nutrients, which can help support liver health.

• The fresh herbs, vegetables, and lemon juice provide antioxidants and anti•inflammatory compounds that can help reduce inflammation in the liver.

• The olive oil provides healthy fats that can help improve cholesterol levels and support liver function.

• The overall low•fat, high•fiber, and nutrient•dense nature of the salad makes it a great choice for seniors with fatty liver disease.

Remember to adjust the seasoning to your taste and enjoy this refreshing and healthy quinoa tabbouleh salad!

54. Turkey and hummus wrap in whole wheat pita

Ingredients:

• 2 whole wheat pita breads, halved
• 1/2 cup hummus
• 4 oz sliced turkey breast
• 1/2 cup shredded lettuce
• 1/4 cup diced cucumber
• 1 tbsp chopped fresh parsley

Instructions:
1. Spread 2•3 tablespoons of hummus inside each pita half.

2. Layer the turkey slices, lettuce, cucumber, and parsley on top of the hummus.

3. Fold the pita in half and enjoy.

This wrap is a great option for a fatty liver diet for seniors for a few reasons:

• Whole wheat pita provides complex carbohydrates, fiber, and B vitamins, which can help support liver health.

• Turkey is a lean protein that is low in saturated fat, which is important for managing fatty liver disease.

• Hummus is a good source of healthy fats from the tahini and olive oil, as well as fiber and protein from the chickpeas.

• The fresh vegetables like lettuce and cucumber provide antioxidants, vitamins, and minerals that can help reduce inflammation in the liver.

This wrap is easy to prepare, portable, and provides a balanced mix of nutrients that can be beneficial for seniors with fatty liver disease. You can also customize the fillings to your taste, such as adding sliced tomatoes, avocado, or a sprinkle of feta cheese.

Remember to choose a high•quality, low•sodium hummus and turkey to keep the sodium content in check. Enjoy this tasty and nutritious wrap as part of a healthy fatty liver diet.

55. Baked yam with steamed green beans

Ingredients:

• 2 medium•sized yams, scrubbed clean
• 1 lb fresh green beans, trimmed
• 1 tbsp olive oil
• Salt and pepper to taste

Instructions:

1. Preheat the oven to 400°F.

2. Pierce the yams several times with a fork. Place them directly on the oven rack and bake for 45•60 minutes, until tender when pierced with a fork.

3. While the yams are baking, bring a medium pot of water to a boil. Add the trimmed green beans and steam for 5•7 minutes, until tender•crisp. Drain and set aside.

4. Once the yams are cooked, remove them from the oven and let cool slightly. Cut them in half lengthwise.

5. Drizzle the yam halves with the olive oil and season with salt and pepper to taste.

6. Serve the baked yams warm, with the steamed green beans on the side.

This dish is an excellent option for a fatty liver diet for seniors for several reasons:

• Yams are a nutrient•dense complex carbohydrate that are high in fiber, vitamins, and minerals. They can help support liver health.

• Green beans are a low•calorie, high•fiber vegetable that provide antioxidants and anti•inflammatory compounds.

• The olive oil adds healthy monounsaturated fats that can help improve cholesterol levels and reduce inflammation.

• The overall meal is low in saturated fat and high in fiber, vitamins, and minerals • all important for managing fatty liver disease.

This simple, yet delicious, baked yam and steamed green bean dish is easy to prepare and can be a great addition to a fatty liver•friendly diet for seniors. Feel free to adjust the seasoning to your taste preferences.

56. Grilled chicken with roasted beets and arugula

Ingredients:

• 4 cups arugula
• 2 tbsp balsamic vinegar
• 1 tbsp Dijon mustard
• 1 tbsp honey

• 4 boneless, skinless chicken breasts
• 1 tbsp olive oil
• 1 tsp dried oregano
• Salt and pepper to taste
• 3 medium beets, peeled and cut into 1•inch cubes
• 2 tbsp olive oil

Instructions:

1. Preheat the oven to 400°F.

2. Toss the beet cubes with 2 tbsp of olive oil and season with salt and pepper. Spread them on a baking sheet and roast for 25•30 minutes, until tender.

3. In the meantime, brush the chicken breasts with 1 tbsp of olive oil and season with oregano, salt, and pepper.

4. Grill the chicken over medium•high heat for 5•7 minutes per side, or until cooked through.

5. In a small bowl, whisk together the balsamic vinegar, Dijon mustard, and honey to make the dressing.

6. In a large bowl, toss the roasted beets and arugula with the dressing. Serve the grilled chicken on top of the beet and arugula salad.

This dish is an excellent option for a fatty liver diet for seniors for several reasons:

• Chicken is a lean protein that is low in saturated fat, which is important for managing fatty liver disease.

• Beets are a nutrient•dense root vegetable that are high in fiber, antioxidants, and anti•inflammatory compounds, which can help support liver health.

• Arugula is a leafy green that is low in calories and high in vitamins, minerals, and antioxidants.

• The olive oil and balsamic vinegar dressing provides healthy fats and anti•inflammatory properties.

• The overall meal is well•balanced, with a focus on lean protein, vegetables, and healthy fats • all important for a fatty liver•friendly diet.

57. Baked trout with lemon and herbs

Ingredients:

- 4 trout fillets (about 4•6 oz each)
- 2 tbsp olive oil
- 2 tbsp fresh lemon juice
- 2 tsp chopped fresh parsley
- 1 tsp chopped fresh dill
- 1 tsp chopped fresh thyme
- Salt and pepper to taste

Instructions:

1. Preheat the oven to 400°F.

2. Place the trout fillets in a baking dish or on a parchment•lined baking sheet.

3. In a small bowl, whisk together the olive oil, lemon juice, parsley, dill, and thyme. Season with salt and pepper.

4. Drizzle the lemon•herb mixture over the trout fillets, making sure to coat them evenly.

5. Bake the trout for 12•15 minutes, or until it flakes easily with a fork. Serve the baked trout warm, with any remaining lemon•herb sauce spooned over the top.

This baked trout dish is an excellent option for a fatty liver diet for seniors for several reasons:

- Trout is a fatty fish that is high in omega•3 fatty acids, which can help reduce inflammation and improve liver function.

- The lemon and herbs provide antioxidants and anti•inflammatory compounds that can also support liver health.

- The overall dish is low in saturated fat and high in protein, which is important for managing fatty liver disease.

- Baking the trout instead of frying it keeps the dish light and healthy.

This simple, yet flavorful, baked trout with lemon and herbs is easy to prepare and can be a great addition to a fatty liver•friendly diet for seniors. Serve it with a side of roasted vegetables or a fresh salad for a complete and nutritious meal.

58. Vegetable lo mein with tofu

Ingredients:

• 8 oz whole wheat lo mein noodles
• 1 tbsp sesame oil
• 1 block (14 oz) firm or extra•firm tofu, cubed
• 2 cups sliced mushrooms
• 1 cup shredded cabbage
• 1 cup sliced bell peppers
• 1 cup sliced carrots
• 2 cloves garlic, minced
• 2 tbsp low•sodium soy sauce
• 1 tbsp rice vinegar
• 1 tsp grated fresh ginger
• 1/4 tsp red pepper flakes (optional)
• Salt and pepper to taste

Instructions:

1. Cook the lo mein noodles according to package instructions. Drain and set aside.

2. In a large skillet or wok, heat the sesame oil over medium•high heat. Add the cubed tofu and cook, stirring occasionally, until lightly browned on all sides, about 5•7 minutes. Remove the tofu from the pan and set aside.

3. In the same pan, add the mushrooms, cabbage, bell peppers, and carrots. Sauté for 5•7 minutes, until the vegetables are tender•crisp.

4. Add the garlic and sauté for an additional minute, until fragrant.

5. Return the cooked tofu to the pan, along with the cooked lo mein noodles, soy sauce, rice vinegar, ginger, and red pepper flakes (if using). Toss everything together until well combined and heated through.

6. Season with salt and pepper to taste. Serve the vegetable lo mein with tofu warm.

This dish is an excellent option for a fatty liver diet for seniors for several reasons:

• Whole wheat lo mein noodles provide complex carbohydrates, fiber, and B vitamins, which can support liver health.

• Tofu is a lean, plant•based protein that is low in saturated fat and can help improve cholesterol levels.

59. Red lentil and vegetable dhal

Ingredients:

- 1 cup red lentils, rinsed
- 4 cups low•sodium vegetable broth
- 1 tbsp olive oil
- 1 onion, diced
- 3 cloves garlic, minced
- 1 tbsp grated fresh ginger
- 1 tsp ground cumin
- 1 tsp ground coriander
- 1/2 tsp turmeric
- 1/4 tsp cayenne pepper (optional)
- 1 cup diced tomatoes
- 1 cup diced carrots
- 1 cup diced cauliflower
- 1 cup baby spinach
- 2 tbsp chopped fresh cilantro
- Salt and pepper to taste

Instructions:

1. In a large pot, combine the rinsed red lentils and vegetable broth. Bring to a boil, then reduce heat and simmer for 15•20 minutes, until the lentils are tender.

2. In a separate skillet, heat the olive oil over medium heat. Add the diced onion and sauté for 3•4 minutes, until translucent.

3. Add the minced garlic, grated ginger, cumin, coriander, turmeric, and cayenne (if using). Sauté for 1 minute, until fragrant.

4. Stir in the diced tomatoes, carrots, and cauliflower. Cook for 5•7 minutes, until the vegetables are tender.

5. Add the cooked lentils and their broth to the vegetable mixture. Stir to combine. Stir in the baby spinach and chopped cilantro. Season with salt and pepper to taste.

6. Serve the red lentil and vegetable dhal warm, over cooked brown rice or quinoa if desired.

This dhal dish is an excellent option for a fatty liver diet for seniors for several reasons:

- Red lentils are a great source of plant•based protein, fiber, and complex carbohydrates, which can help support liver health.

- The variety of vegetables, such as carrots, cauliflower, and spinach, provide antioxidants, vitamins, and minerals that can help reduce inflammation in the liver.

- The spices, like cumin, coriander, and turmeric, have anti•inflammatory properties that can also benefit the liver.

60. Whole wheat spaghetti with marinara and sautéed zucchini

Ingredients:

• 2 tbsp tomato paste
• 1 tsp dried oregano
• 1/2 tsp dried basil
• Salt and pepper to taste
• Grated Parmesan cheese (optional)

• 8 oz whole wheat spaghetti
• 1 tbsp olive oil
• 2 medium zucchini, sliced into half•moons
• 3 cloves garlic, minced
• 1 (28 oz) can crushed tomatoes

Instructions:

1. Bring a large pot of salted water to a boil. Cook the whole wheat spaghetti according to package instructions until al dente. Drain and set aside.

2. In a large skillet, heat the olive oil over medium heat. Add the sliced zucchini and sauté for 5•7 minutes, until tender and lightly browned.

3. Add the minced garlic to the skillet and sauté for an additional minute, until fragrant.

4. Pour in the crushed tomatoes and tomato paste. Stir in the dried oregano and basil. Season with salt and pepper to taste.

5. Reduce the heat to low and let the marinara sauce simmer for 10•15 minutes, stirring occasionally, to allow the flavors to meld.

6. Add the cooked whole wheat spaghetti to the skillet with the marinara sauce and toss to coat the noodles evenly. Serve the whole wheat spaghetti with marinara and sautéed zucchini warm, with a sprinkle of grated Parmesan cheese on top, if desired.

This dish is an excellent option for a fatty liver diet for seniors for several reasons:

• Whole wheat spaghetti provides complex carbohydrates, fiber, and B vitamins, which can support liver health.

• Zucchini is a low•calorie, high•fiber vegetable that provides antioxidants and anti•inflammatory compounds.

• The marinara sauce is a good source of lycopene, an antioxidant that can help protect the liver.

• The overall dish is low in saturated fat and high in fiber, vitamins, and minerals • all important for managing fatty liver disease

61. Overnight chia pudding with berries

Ingredients:

- 1/4 cup chia seeds
- 1 cup unsweetened almond milk (or milk of your choice)
- 1 tbsp maple syrup (or honey)
- 1/2 tsp vanilla extract
- 1 cup mixed berries (such as blueberries, raspberries, and/or blackberries)

Instructions:

1. In a medium•sized bowl, whisk together the chia seeds, almond milk, maple syrup, and vanilla extract until well combined.

2. Cover the bowl and refrigerate for at least 4 hours, or overnight.

3. When ready to serve, give the chia pudding a stir to incorporate any thickened chia seeds. Top the chia pudding with the mixed berries.

This overnight chia pudding with berries is an excellent option for a fatty liver diet for seniors for several reasons:

- Chia seeds are a great source of fiber, protein, and omega•3 fatty acids, which can help support liver health.

- Berries are high in antioxidants, vitamins, and fiber, which can help reduce inflammation in the liver.

- The almond milk provides a dairy•free, low•fat option that is easy to digest.

- The maple syrup or honey adds a touch of sweetness without excessive added sugar.

- The overall dish is low in saturated fat, high in fiber, and packed with nutrients that are beneficial for managing fatty liver disease.

This overnight chia pudding with berries is a simple, make•ahead breakfast or snack that can be a great addition to a fatty liver•friendly diet for seniors. It's easy to prepare, portable, and can be customized with your favorite berries or other toppings, such as chopped nuts or a sprinkle of cinnamon.

Remember to adjust the sweetener to your taste preferences, and enjoy this delicious and liver•supporting chia pudding.

62. Frittata with spinach, tomatoes, and feta

Ingredients:

• 8 large eggs
• 1/4 cup unsweetened almond milk (or milk of your choice)
• 2 cups fresh spinach, chopped
• 1 cup cherry tomatoes, halved
• 1/2 cup crumbled feta cheese
• 1 tbsp olive oil
• 1 clove garlic, minced
• Salt and pepper to taste

Instructions:

1. Preheat your oven to 375°F.

2. In a large bowl, whisk together the eggs and almond milk. Season with a pinch of salt and pepper.

3. In a 9•inch oven•safe skillet, heat the olive oil over medium heat. Add the minced garlic and sauté for 1 minute, until fragrant.

4. Add the chopped spinach to the skillet and sauté for 2•3 minutes, until the spinach is wilted. Pour the egg mixture over the spinach, then top with the halved cherry tomatoes and crumbled feta cheese.

5. Transfer the skillet to the preheated oven and bake for 18•22 minutes, or until the frittata is set and the edges are lightly browned. Remove the frittata from the oven and let it cool for a few minutes before slicing and serving.

This spinach, tomato, and feta frittata is an excellent option for a fatty liver diet for seniors for several reasons:

• Eggs are a high•quality protein that can help support liver function. Spinach is a nutrient•dense leafy green that provides antioxidants and anti•inflammatory compounds.

• Cherry tomatoes are a good source of lycopene, an antioxidant that can help protect the liver. Feta cheese is a low•fat, high•protein dairy option that can add flavor and nutrients to the dish.

• The overall dish Is low in saturated fat and high in fiber, vitamins, and minerals • all important for managing fatty liver disease.

63. Plain Greek yogurt with fresh fruit and nuts

Ingredients:

• 1 cup plain, unsweetened Greek yogurt
• 1 cup mixed fresh fruit (such as berries, sliced peaches, or diced mango)
• 2 tbsp chopped walnuts or almonds

Instructions:

1. Scoop the plain Greek yogurt into a bowl.

2. Top the yogurt with the mixed fresh fruit.

3. Sprinkle the chopped nuts over the fruit. Serve immediately.

This simple dish is an excellent option for a fatty liver diet for seniors for several reasons:

• Greek yogurt is a great source of protein, which can help support liver function. It's also low in fat and contains probiotics that can benefit gut health.

• Fresh fruits like berries, peaches, and mango are high in fiber, vitamins, and antioxidants that can help reduce inflammation in the liver.

• Nuts, such as walnuts and almonds, provide healthy fats, fiber, and anti•inflammatory compounds that can also support liver health.

• The overall dish is low in added sugars and high in nutrients that are important for managing fatty liver disease.

This plain Greek yogurt with fresh fruit and nuts is a quick, easy, and nutritious option that can be enjoyed for breakfast, a snack, or even dessert. It's versatile, so you can use your favorite seasonal fruits and nuts.

Remember to choose plain, unsweetened Greek yogurt to keep the sugar content low. You can also adjust the portion sizes to your liking. Enjoy this delicious and liver•supporting dish!

64. Whole grain toast with mashed avocado

Ingredients:

• 2 slices of whole grain bread
• 1 ripe avocado, mashed
• 1 tbsp lemon juice
• 1/4 tsp garlic powder (optional)
• Salt and pepper to taste

Instructions:

1. Toast the whole grain bread until lightly golden brown.

2. In a small bowl, mash the avocado with a fork. Stir in the lemon juice, garlic powder (if using), and a pinch of salt and pepper.

3. Spread the mashed avocado evenly over the toasted whole grain bread slices.

4. Serve the whole grain toast with mashed avocado immediately.

This dish is an excellent option for a fatty liver diet for seniors for several reasons:

• Whole grain bread provides complex carbohydrates, fiber, and B vitamins, which can support liver health.

• Avocado is a great source of healthy monounsaturated fats, which can help improve cholesterol levels and reduce inflammation in the liver.

• The lemon juice adds a touch of acidity and vitamin C, which can also have anti•inflammatory benefits.

• The overall dish is low in saturated fat and high in fiber, healthy fats, and nutrients • all important for managing fatty liver disease.

This whole grain toast with mashed avocado is a simple, yet nutritious, option that can be enjoyed for breakfast, a snack, or even a light lunch. It's easy to prepare and can be customized with additional toppings, such as a sprinkle of red pepper flakes or a drizzle of olive oil, if desired.

Remember to choose a high•quality, whole grain bread and a ripe, creamy avocado for the best flavor and texture. Enjoy this delicious and liver•supporting dish!

65. Green smoothie with kale, mango, and coconut water

Ingredients:

• 1 cup packed kale leaves, stems removed
• 1 cup frozen mango chunks
• 1 cup unsweetened coconut water
• 1/2 cup plain, unsweetened almond milk (or milk of your choice)
• 1 tbsp ground flaxseed (optional)
• 1 tsp honey (optional)

Instructions:
1. Add the kale, frozen mango, coconut water, and almond milk to a high•powered blender.

2. Blend on high speed until the mixture is smooth and creamy, about 1•2 minutes.

3. If using, add the ground flaxseed and honey, and blend again briefly to incorporate. Pour the green smoothie into a glass and enjoy immediately.

This green smoothie is an excellent option for a fatty liver diet for seniors for several reasons:

• Kale is a nutrient•dense leafy green that is high in antioxidants, vitamins, and minerals, which can help support liver health.

• Mango is a sweet, tropical fruit that is rich in vitamins, fiber, and anti•inflammatory compounds.

• Coconut water provides hydration and electrolytes without added sugars or artificial ingredients.

• Almond milk is a dairy•free, low•fat option that can add creaminess to the smoothie.

• Ground flaxseed is a good source of omega•3 fatty acids, which can help reduce inflammation in the liver.

• The overall smoothie is low in saturated fat, high in fiber, and packed with nutrients that are beneficial for managing fatty liver disease.

This green smoothie is a refreshing and nutritious way to start the day or enjoy as a snack. The combination of kale, mango, and coconut water provides a delicious and liver•supporting flavor profile.

66. Roasted Brussels sprouts with balsamic glaze

Ingredients:

• 1 lb Brussels sprouts, trimmed and halved
• 2 tbsp olive oil
• Salt and pepper to taste
• 2 tbsp balsamic vinegar
• 1 tbsp honey

Instructions:
1. Preheat your oven to 400°F.

2. In a large bowl, toss the trimmed and halved Brussels sprouts with the olive oil. Season with a pinch of salt and pepper.

3. Spread the Brussels sprouts in a single layer on a baking sheet. Roast for 20•25 minutes, tossing halfway, until the sprouts are tender and lightly browned.

4. In a small saucepan, combine the balsamic vinegar and honey. Bring the mixture to a simmer over medium heat, stirring occasionally, until it thickens into a glaze, about 5 minutes.

5. Remove the roasted Brussels sprouts from the oven and transfer them to a serving bowl. Drizzle the balsamic glaze over the top and toss gently to coat. Serve the roasted Brussels sprouts with balsamic glaze warm.

This dish is an excellent option for a fatty liver diet for seniors for several reasons:

• Brussels sprouts are a cruciferous vegetable that are high in fiber, vitamins, and antioxidants, which can help support liver health.
• The balsamic vinegar provides a tangy, flavorful glaze that is low in added sugars.
• The honey adds a touch of sweetness without excessive sugar content.
• The overall dish is low in saturated fat and high in fiber, vitamins, and anti•inflammatory compounds • all important for managing fatty liver disease.

Roasted Brussels sprouts with a balsamic glaze is a simple, yet delicious, side dish that can be enjoyed by seniors with fatty liver disease. The combination of the caramelized Brussels sprouts and the sweet•tart balsamic glaze creates a flavorful and liver•supporting meal.

Feel free to adjust the amount of honey to your taste preferences. Enjoy this nutritious and liver•friendly roasted Brussels sprouts dish!

67. Sautéed Swiss chard with garlic and lemon

Ingredients:

• 1 lb Swiss chard, stems removed and leaves chopped
• 1 tbsp olive oil
• 3 cloves garlic, minced
• 1 tbsp lemon juice
• Salt and pepper to taste

Instructions:

1. In a large skillet, heat the olive oil over medium heat.

2. Add the minced garlic and sauté for 1•2 minutes, until fragrant.

3. Add the chopped Swiss chard leaves to the skillet. Sauté for 5•7 minutes, stirring occasionally, until the chard is wilted and tender.

4. Remove the skillet from the heat and stir in the lemon juice. Season with salt and pepper to taste. Serve the sautéed Swiss chard warm.

This dish is an excellent option for a fatty liver diet for seniors for several reasons:

• Swiss chard is a nutrient•dense leafy green that is high in vitamins, minerals, and antioxidants, which can help support liver health.

• The garlic provides anti•inflammatory properties that can also benefit the liver.

• Lemon juice adds a bright, tangy flavor while providing vitamin C, which has antioxidant effects.

• The overall dish is low in saturated fat and high in fiber, vitamins, and minerals • all important for managing fatty liver disease.

Sautéed Swiss chard with garlic and lemon is a simple, yet flavorful, side dish that can be a great addition to a fatty liver•friendly diet for seniors. The chard cooks down quickly, making it an easy and convenient option.

Feel free to adjust the amount of lemon juice or garlic to your taste preferences. You can also serve the sautéed Swiss chard as a main dish, paired with a lean protein and a whole grain for a complete and liver•supporting meal.

68. Baked carrot fries

Ingredients:

• 1 lb carrots, peeled and cut into 1/4•inch thick fry•shaped pieces
• 1 tbsp olive oil
• 1 tsp paprika
• 1/2 tsp garlic powder
• 1/4 tsp salt
• 1/4 tsp black pepper

Instructions:

1. Preheat your oven to 400°F. Line a baking sheet with parchment paper.

2. In a large bowl, toss the carrot fry pieces with the olive oil, paprika, garlic powder, salt, and pepper until evenly coated.

3. Spread the carrot fries in a single layer on the prepared baking sheet.

4. Bake for 20•25 minutes, flipping the fries halfway through, until they are tender and lightly browned. Serve the baked carrot fries warm.

This dish is an excellent option for a fatty liver diet for seniors for several reasons:

• Carrots are a nutrient•dense vegetable that are high in fiber, vitamins, and antioxidants, which can help support liver health.

• Baking the carrot fries instead of frying them keeps the dish low in saturated fat and calories.

• The spices, like paprika and garlic powder, add flavor without the need for excessive salt or sugar.

• The overall dish is low in saturated fat and high in fiber, vitamins, and minerals • all important for managing fatty liver disease.

Baked carrot fries are a healthy and delicious alternative to traditional potato fries. They can be enjoyed as a side dish or a snack, and they're easy to prepare.

Feel free to experiment with different seasoning blends to find the flavors you enjoy most. Enjoy these nutritious and liver•supporting baked carrot fries!

69. Wild rice pilaf with mushrooms and peas

Ingredients:

- 1 cup uncooked wild rice
- 2 cups low•sodium vegetable or chicken broth
- 1 tbsp olive oil
- 8 oz sliced mushrooms
- 1 cup frozen peas
- 2 cloves garlic, minced
- 1 tsp dried thyme
- Salt and pepper to taste

Instructions:

1. In a medium saucepan, combine the wild rice and broth. Bring to a boil, then reduce heat, cover, and simmer for 45•50 minutes, until the rice is tender and the liquid is absorbed.

2. In a large skillet, heat the olive oil over medium heat. Add the sliced mushrooms and sauté for 5•7 minutes, until they are tender and lightly browned.

3. Add the minced garlic and dried thyme to the skillet. Sauté for 1 minute, until fragrant.

4. Stir in the cooked wild rice and frozen peas. Cook for an additional 2•3 minutes, until the peas are heated through.

5. Season the wild rice pilaf with salt and pepper to taste. Serve the wild rice pilaf with mushrooms and peas warm.

This dish is an excellent option for a fatty liver diet for seniors for several reasons:
• Wild rice is a whole grain that is high in fiber, protein, and B vitamins, which can support liver health.

• Mushrooms are a nutrient•dense vegetable that provide antioxidants and anti•inflammatory compounds. Peas are a good source of fiber, vitamins, and minerals that can also benefit the liver.

• The overall dish is low in saturated fat and high in fiber, protein, and nutrients • all important for managing fatty liver disease.

This wild rice pilaf with mushrooms and peas is a flavorful and nutritious side dish that can be a great addition to a fatty liver•friendly diet for seniors. It's easy to prepare and can be served as a main dish or alongside a lean protein for a complete meal.

70. Roasted cauliflower with turmeric

Ingredients:

• 1 head of cauliflower, cut into florets
• 2 tbsp olive oil
• 1 tsp ground turmeric
• 1/2 tsp ground cumin
• 1/4 tsp garlic powder
• Salt and pepper to taste

Instructions:

1. Preheat your oven to 400°F. Line a baking sheet with parchment paper.

2. In a large bowl, toss the cauliflower florets with the olive oil, turmeric, cumin, garlic powder, and a pinch of salt and pepper until the cauliflower is evenly coated.

3. Spread the seasoned cauliflower in a single layer on the prepared baking sheet.

4. Roast the cauliflower for 20•25 minutes, flipping halfway, until it is tender and lightly browned. Remove the roasted cauliflower from the oven and serve warm.

This roasted cauliflower with turmeric dish is an excellent option for a fatty liver diet for seniors for several reasons:

• Cauliflower is a cruciferous vegetable that is high in fiber, vitamins, and antioxidants, which can help support liver health.

• Turmeric is a spice with potent anti•inflammatory properties that can also benefit the liver.

• The cumin and garlic add flavor without the need for excessive salt or sugar.

• The overall dish is low in saturated fat and high in fiber, vitamins, and anti•inflammatory compounds • all important for managing fatty liver disease.

Roasted cauliflower with turmeric is a simple, yet flavorful, side dish that can be a great addition to a fatty liver•friendly diet for seniors. The combination of the tender, caramelized cauliflower and the warm spices creates a delicious and nutritious meal.

Feel free to adjust the seasoning to your taste preferences. You can also try adding other herbs or spices, such as paprika or chili powder, to vary the flavor profile.

71. Fresh fruit salsa

Ingredients:

• 1 cup diced mango
• 1 cup diced pineapple
• 1 cup diced strawberries
• 1/2 cup diced red onion
• 1/4 cup chopped fresh cilantro
• 2 tbsp lime juice
• 1 tsp grated lime zest
• 1/4 tsp ground cumin
• Salt and pepper to taste

Instructions:
1. In a medium bowl, combine the diced mango, pineapple, strawberries, and red onion.

2. Add the chopped cilantro, lime juice, lime zest, and ground cumin. Stir gently to mix.

3. Season the fruit salsa with salt and pepper to taste.

4. Cover and refrigerate for at least 30 minutes to allow the flavors to meld.

5. Serve the fresh fruit salsa chilled, with whole grain crackers, grilled chicken, or fish.

This fresh fruit salsa is an excellent option for a fatty liver diet for seniors for several reasons:

• The variety of fruits, such as mango, pineapple, and strawberries, provide a range of vitamins, minerals, and antioxidants that can help support liver health.
• The red onion and cilantro add anti•inflammatory properties to the salsa.
• The lime juice and zest provide a bright, tangy flavor without the need for added sugars.
• The overall dish is low in saturated fat and high in fiber, vitamins, and anti•inflammatory compounds • all important for managing fatty liver disease.

This fresh fruit salsa is a versatile and flavorful option that can be enjoyed as a dip, a topping for grilled proteins, or even as a refreshing side dish. It's easy to prepare and can be a great way to incorporate more nutrient•dense fruits into a fatty liver•friendly diet for seniors.

Feel free to adjust the ingredient ratios or swap in your favorite seasonal fruits to suit your taste preferences. Enjoy this delicious and liver•supporting fresh fruit salsa!

72. Roasted chickpeas

Ingredients:

• 1 (15 oz) can of chickpeas, drained and rinsed
• 1 tbsp olive oil
• 1 tsp ground cumin
• 1/2 tsp garlic powder
• 1/4 tsp paprika
• 1/4 tsp salt
• 1/4 tsp black pepper

Instructions:
1. Preheat your oven to 400°F. Line a baking sheet with parchment paper.

2. Pat the drained and rinsed chickpeas dry with a paper towel or clean kitchen towel.

3. In a medium bowl, toss the chickpeas with the olive oil, cumin, garlic powder, paprika, salt, and pepper until they are evenly coated.

4. Spread the seasoned chickpeas in a single layer on the prepared baking sheet.

5. Roast the chickpeas for 20•25 minutes, shaking the pan halfway, until they are crispy and lightly browned.

6. Remove the roasted chickpeas from the oven and let them cool for a few minutes before serving.

This roasted chickpea recipe is an excellent option for a fatty liver diet for seniors for several reasons:

• Chickpeas are a good source of plant•based protein, fiber, and complex carbohydrates, which can help support liver health.
• The spices, like cumin, garlic, and paprika, add flavor without the need for excessive salt or sugar.
• Roasting the chickpeas gives them a crispy texture, making them a satisfying and crunchy snack.
• The overall dish is low in saturated fat and high in fiber, protein, and nutrients • all important for managing fatty liver disease.

Roasted chickpeas can be enjoyed as a snack, added to salads or bowls, or used as a crunchy topping for soups and stews. They are a versatile and liver•supporting option that can be a great addition to a fatty liver diet for seniors.

73. Black bean and corn salad

Ingredients:

- 1 (15 oz) can black beans, drained and rinsed
- 1 (15 oz) can corn, drained
- 1 cup diced tomatoes
- 1/2 cup diced red onion
- 1/4 cup chopped fresh cilantro
- 2 tbsp lime juice
- 1 tbsp olive oil
- 1 tsp ground cumin
- 1/4 tsp chili powder
- Salt and pepper to taste

Instructions:
1. In a large bowl, combine the drained and rinsed black beans, drained corn, diced tomatoes, and diced red onion.

2. Add the chopped cilantro, lime juice, olive oil, cumin, and chili powder. Stir to mix everything together.

3. Season the salad with salt and pepper to taste. Cover and refrigerate for at least 30 minutes to allow the flavors to meld. Serve the black bean and corn salad chilled or at room temperature.

This black bean and corn salad is an excellent option for a fatty liver diet for seniors for several reasons:
- Black beans are a good source of plant•based protein, fiber, and complex carbohydrates, which can help support liver health. Corn provides additional fiber and nutrients.

- The tomatoes, red onion, and cilantro add antioxidants and anti•inflammatory compounds.

- The lime juice and spices, like cumin and chili powder, add flavor without the need for excessive salt or sugar. The overall dish is low in saturated fat and high in fiber, protein, and nutrients • all important for managing fatty liver disease.

This black bean and corn salad is a refreshing and flavorful side dish or light meal that can be a great addition to a fatty liver•friendly diet for seniors. It's easy to prepare and can be made in advance, making it a convenient option.

74. Guacamole with veggie sticks

Ingredients:

- 2 ripe avocados, pitted and mashed
- 2 tbsp diced red onion
- 1 tbsp lime juice
- 2 tsp chopped fresh cilantro
- 1/4 tsp ground cumin
- Salt and pepper to taste
- Assorted raw vegetable sticks (such as carrot, celery, cucumber, bell pepper)

Instructions:

1. In a medium bowl, mash the avocados with a fork or potato masher until they reach your desired consistency.

2. Stir in the diced red onion, lime juice, chopped cilantro, and ground cumin. Season with salt and pepper to taste. Serve the guacamole immediately with the assorted raw vegetable sticks for dipping.

This guacamole with veggie sticks is an excellent option for a fatty liver diet for seniors for several reasons:

- Avocados are a great source of healthy monounsaturated fats, which can help improve cholesterol levels and reduce inflammation in the liver.

- The fresh vegetables, such as carrots, celery, and bell peppers, provide a variety of vitamins, minerals, and antioxidants that can support liver health.

- The lime juice, cilantro, and onion add flavor and anti•inflammatory properties to the guacamole.

- The overall dish is low in saturated fat and high in fiber, healthy fats, and nutrients • all important for managing fatty liver disease.

Guacamole is a versatile and nutrient•dense dip that can be enjoyed as a snack or as part of a larger meal. Pairing it with a variety of raw vegetable sticks makes it a liver•friendly and satisfying option for seniors.

Feel free to adjust the seasoning to your taste preferences. You can also try adding other ingredients, such as diced tomatoes or jalapeño, to customize the guacamole to your liking.

75. Egg salad lettuce wraps

Ingredients:

• 6 hard•boiled eggs, peeled and chopped
• 2 tbsp plain Greek yogurt
• 1 tbsp Dijon mustard
• 1 tbsp chopped fresh dill (or 1 tsp dried dill)
• 1 tbsp lemon juice
• Salt and pepper to taste
• 8•10 large lettuce leaves (such as romaine or butter lettuce)

Instructions:

1. In a medium bowl, combine the chopped hard•boiled eggs, Greek yogurt, Dijon mustard, fresh dill (or dried dill), and lemon juice. Stir until well mixed.

2. Season the egg salad with salt and pepper to taste.

3. Lay the lettuce leaves flat on a clean surface. Scoop a portion of the egg salad onto the center of each lettuce leaf. Fold the sides of the lettuce leaf over the egg salad and serve.

This egg salad lettuce wrap recipe is an excellent option for a fatty liver diet for seniors for several reasons:

• Eggs are a high•quality protein that can help support liver function.• The Greek yogurt provides additional protein and probiotics, which can benefit gut health.

• The fresh dill and lemon juice add flavor and anti•inflammatory properties to the egg salad.

• Serving the egg salad in lettuce wraps instead of bread or crackers keeps the dish low in carbohydrates and calories.

• The overall dish is low in saturated fat and high in protein, vitamins, and minerals • all important for managing fatty liver disease.

Egg salad lettuce wraps are a simple, yet satisfying, option that can be enjoyed for a light lunch or snack. They are easy to prepare and can be customized with your favorite herbs, spices, or additional vegetables.

Feel free to adjust the amount of yogurt or seasonings to suit your taste preferences. Enjoy these nutritious and liver•supporting egg salad lettuce wraps!

76. Grilled tuna with mango salsa

Ingredients:

For the Mango Salsa:
• 1 ripe mango, diced
• 1/2 cup diced red onion
• 1/4 cup chopped fresh cilantro
• 1 tbsp lime juice
• 1/4 tsp ground cumin
• Salt and pepper to taste

For the Tuna:
• 4 (4•6 oz) tuna steaks
• 1 tbsp olive oil
• Salt and pepper to taste

Instructions:

1. Make the mango salsa: In a medium bowl, combine the diced mango, red onion, cilantro, lime juice, and cumin. Season with salt and pepper to taste. Cover and refrigerate until ready to serve.

2. Prepare the tuna: Preheat your grill or grill pan to medium•high heat. Brush the tuna steaks with the olive oil and season with salt and pepper.

3. Grill the tuna for 2•3 minutes per side, or until it reaches your desired doneness. Be careful not to overcook. Serve the grilled tuna steaks topped with the chilled mango salsa.

This grilled tuna with mango salsa dish is an excellent option for a fatty liver diet for seniors for several reasons:

• Tuna is a fatty fish that is high in omega•3 fatty acids, which can help reduce inflammation in the liver.
• Mango is a sweet, tropical fruit that is rich in vitamins, fiber, and antioxidants.
• The fresh cilantro, lime juice, and cumin in the salsa add anti•inflammatory properties.
• The overall dish is low in saturated fat and high in protein, healthy fats, and nutrients • all important for managing fatty liver disease.

Grilled tuna with mango salsa is a flavorful and nutritious meal that can be a great addition to a fatty liver•friendly diet for seniors. The sweetness of the mango pairs beautlfully with the savory tuna, and the salsa adds a refreshing and vibrant element to the dish.

77. White bean and kale soup

Ingredients:

• 1 tbsp olive oil
• 1 onion, diced
• 3 cloves garlic, minced
• 1 tsp dried thyme
• 1 tsp dried oregano
• 4 cups low•sodium vegetable or chicken broth
• 1 (15 oz) can white beans, drained and rinsed
• 4 cups chopped kale, stems removed
• Salt and pepper to taste

Instructions:

1. In a large pot or Dutch oven, heat the olive oil over medium heat. Add the diced onion and sauté for 3•4 minutes, until translucent.

2. Add the minced garlic, dried thyme, and dried oregano. Sauté for 1 minute, until fragrant.

3. Pour in the low•sodium broth and add the drained and rinsed white beans. Bring the soup to a simmer.

4. Stir in the chopped kale and let the soup simmer for 10•15 minutes, until the kale is tender. Season the white bean and kale soup with salt and pepper to taste. Serve the soup warm.

This white bean and kale soup is an excellent option for a fatty liver diet for seniors for several reasons:

• White beans are a good source of plant•based protein, fiber, and complex carbohydrates, which can help support liver health.

• Kale is a nutrient•dense leafy green that is high in vitamins, minerals, and antioxidants, which can also benefit the liver.

• The herbs, like thyme and oregano, add flavor without the need for excessive sodium or fat.

• The overall soup is low in saturated fat and high in fiber, protein, and nutrients • all important for managing fatty liver disease.

78. Lentil and bulgur salad

Ingredients:

• 1 cup cooked lentils
• 1/2 cup cooked bulgur
• 1/2 cup diced cucumber
• 1/4 cup diced tomatoes
• 2 tbsp chopped parsley
• 2 tbsp lemon juice
• 1 tbsp olive oil
• 1 tsp ground cumin
• Salt and pepper to taste

Instructions:

1. In a medium bowl, combine the cooked lentils, bulgur, cucumber, tomatoes, and parsley.

2. In a small bowl, whisk together the lemon juice, olive oil, cumin, salt, and pepper. Pour the dressing over the lentil and bulgur mixture and toss gently to coat. Serve chilled or at room temperature.

This salad is a great option for a fatty liver diet for seniors for a few reasons:

1. Lentils are a good source of plant•based protein, fiber, and complex carbohydrates, which can help support liver health.

2. Bulgur is a whole grain that is high in fiber and can help promote feelings of fullness.

3. The vegetables, herbs, and healthy fats from the olive oil provide antioxidants and anti•inflammatory nutrients that can help reduce inflammation in the liver.

The lemon juice and cumin also add flavor without the need for excessive salt, which is important for managing blood pressure and fluid retention, common issues for those with fatty liver disease.

This salad can be a nutritious and satisfying side dish or light main course for seniors following a fatty liver diet.

79. Curried turkey lettuce cups

Ingredients:

- 1 lb ground turkey
- 1 tbsp olive oil
- 1 onion, diced
- 2 cloves garlic, minced
- 1 tbsp curry powder
- 1 tsp ground cumin
- 1/2 tsp ground coriander
- 1/4 tsp cayenne pepper (optional)
- 1 cup diced tomatoes
- 1/4 cup low•sodium chicken or vegetable broth
- Salt and pepper to taste
- 12•16 large lettuce leaves (such as romaine or bibb)
- Chopped cilantro for garnish (optional)

Instructions:

1. In a large skillet, heat the olive oil over medium heat. Add the ground turkey and cook, breaking it up with a wooden spoon, until browned, about 5•7 minutes.

2. Add the onion and garlic and cook for 2•3 minutes until fragrant.

3. Stir in the curry powder, cumin, coriander, and cayenne (if using). Cook for 1 minute to toast the spices.

4. Add the diced tomatoes and broth. Simmer for 5•10 minutes, until the liquid has reduced and the flavors have melded.

5. Season with salt and pepper to taste. Spoon the curried turkey mixture into the lettuce leaves. Garnish with chopped cilantro if desired.

This dish is a great option for a fatty liver diet for seniors for a few reasons:

1. Ground turkey is a lean protein source that is lower in saturated fat compared to red meat.

2. The spices, such as curry powder and cumin, provide anti•inflammatory benefits.

3. The lettuce cups provide a low•calorie, high•fiber vehicle for the turkey mixture.

4. The dish is easy to prepare and can be a satisfying main course or appetizer.

80. Loaded baked potato with broccoli, salsa

Ingredients:

• 4 medium russet potatoes
• 1 cup steamed broccoli florets
• 1/2 cup low•fat plain Greek yogurt
• 2 tbsp grated low•fat cheddar cheese
• 1/4 cup fresh salsa
• 2 tbsp chopped green onions
• Salt and pepper to taste

Instructions:
1. Preheat the oven to 400°F. Scrub the potatoes and prick them several times with a fork. Bake for 50•60 minutes, until tender when pierced with a fork.

2. Remove the potatoes from the oven and let cool for 5 minutes. Slice each potato in half lengthwise.

3. Scoop out the flesh of the potatoes into a bowl, leaving a thin layer of potato attached to the skin.

4. Mash the potato flesh with a fork or potato masher. Stir in the Greek yogurt, 1 tbsp of the cheddar cheese, salt, and pepper. Spoon the mashed potato mixture back into the potato skins.

5. Top each potato half with the steamed broccoli florets, the remaining 1 tbsp of cheddar cheese, the salsa, and the chopped green onions. Serve immediately.

This loaded baked potato dish is a great option for a fatty liver diet for seniors for a few reasons:

1. Potatoes are a complex carbohydrate that can provide sustained energy without spiking blood sugar levels.

2. Broccoli is a cruciferous vegetable that is high in fiber and antioxidants, which can help support liver health.

3. The Greek yogurt provides protein and probiotics, which can aid digestion and reduce inflammation. The salsa adds flavor and antioxidants without the need for excessive salt or fat.

81. Grilled chicken kabobs with vegetables

Ingredients:

- 1 lb boneless, skinless chicken breasts, cut into 1•inch cubes
- 1 red bell pepper, cut into 1•inch pieces
- 1 yellow bell pepper, cut into 1•inch pieces
- 1 zucchini, cut into 1•inch pieces
- 1 red onion, cut into 1•inch pieces
- 2 tbsp olive oil
- 2 tsp dried oregano
- 1 tsp garlic powder
- 1/2 tsp paprika
- Salt and pepper to taste

Instructions:

1. In a large bowl, combine the chicken, bell peppers, zucchini, and onion. Drizzle with the olive oil and sprinkle with the oregano, garlic powder, paprika, salt, and pepper. Toss to coat the ingredients evenly.

2. Thread the chicken and vegetables onto metal or wooden skewers, alternating the ingredients. Preheat the grill to medium•high heat.

3. Grill the kabobs for 12•15 minutes, turning occasionally, until the chicken is cooked through and the vegetables are tender. Serve the grilled chicken kabobs immediately.

This dish is an excellent choice for a fatty liver diet for seniors for several reasons:

1. Chicken is a lean protein source that is low in saturated fat, which is important for managing fatty liver disease.

2. The variety of vegetables, including bell peppers, zucchini, and onions, provide fiber, vitamins, and antioxidants that can support liver health.

3. The spices, such as oregano and paprika, have anti•inflammatory properties that can help reduce inflammation in the liver.

4. Grilling the kabobs is a healthy cooking method that doesn't require added oils or fats.

The combination of lean protein, fiber•rich vegetables, and anti•inflammatory spices makes this a nutritious and liver•friendly meal for seniors following a fatty liver diet.

82. Baked haddock with tomatoes and herbs

Ingredients:

• 1 lb haddock fillets
• 2 cups diced tomatoes (fresh or canned, no•salt•added)
• 1/4 cup chopped fresh parsley
• 2 tbsp chopped fresh basil
• 2 cloves garlic, minced
• 1 tbsp olive oil
• 1/4 tsp salt
• 1/4 tsp black pepper

Instructions:

1. Preheat the oven to 400°F.

2. In a baking dish, arrange the haddock fillets in a single layer.

3. In a small bowl, combine the diced tomatoes, parsley, basil, garlic, olive oil, salt, and pepper. Mix well.

4. Spoon the tomato mixture over the haddock fillets, making sure to distribute it evenly.

5. Bake for 15•20 minutes, or until the fish is opaque and flakes easily with a fork. Serve the baked haddock immediately.

This dish is an excellent choice for a fatty liver diet for seniors for several reasons:

1. Haddock is a lean, white fish that is low in mercury and high in omega•3 fatty acids, which can help reduce inflammation in the liver.

2. Tomatoes are a good source of lycopene, an antioxidant that has been shown to have protective effects on the liver.

3. The fresh herbs, such as parsley and basil, provide additional antioxidants and anti•inflammatory properties.

4. The dish is baked, which is a healthier cooking method compared to frying, and it doesn't require the addition of excessive amounts of oil or butter.

The combination of lean protein, nutrient•dense vegetables, and healthy cooking methods makes this baked haddock dish a great option for seniors following a fatty liver diet.

83. Veggie fried cauliflower rice

Ingredients:

• 1 head of cauliflower, riced (about 4 cups riced cauliflower)
• 1 tbsp olive oil
• 1 onion, diced
• 2 cloves garlic, minced
• 1 cup diced bell peppers (any color)
• 1 cup diced mushrooms
• 1 cup frozen peas
• 2 tbsp low•sodium soy sauce or tamari
• 1 tsp sesame oil
• Salt and pepper to taste
• Chopped green onions for garnish (optional)

Instructions:

1. In a food processor, pulse the cauliflower florets until they resemble rice•sized grains. Set aside.

2. In a large skillet or wok, heat the olive oil over medium•high heat. Add the onion and garlic and sauté for 2•3 minutes until fragrant.

3. Add the riced cauliflower, bell peppers, mushrooms, and frozen peas to the skillet. Sauté for 5•7 minutes, stirring frequently, until the vegetables are tender.

4. Stir in the soy sauce or tamari and sesame oil. Season with salt and pepper to taste. Serve the veggie fried cauliflower rice hot, garnished with chopped green onions if desired.

This dish is an excellent choice for a fatty liver diet for seniors for several reasons:

1. Cauliflower is a low•carb, high•fiber vegetable that can help support liver health.

2. The variety of vegetables, including bell peppers, mushrooms, and peas, provide a range of vitamins, minerals, and antioxidants that can help reduce inflammation in the liver.

3. The dish is low in calories and fat, making it a suitable option for seniors who need to manage their weight and blood sugar levels.

4. The soy sauce or tamari provides a savory flavor without the need for excessive salt, which is important for managing blood pressure and fluid retention.

84. Split pea and vegetable soup

Ingredients:

• 1 cup dried split peas, rinsed
• 6 cups low•sodium vegetable or chicken broth
• 1 tbsp olive oil
• 1 onion, diced
• 2 carrots, peeled and diced
• 2 celery stalks, diced
• 3 cloves garlic, minced
• 1 tsp dried thyme
• 1/2 tsp ground cumin
• Salt and pepper to taste
• Chopped parsley for garnish (optional)

Instructions:
1. In a large pot, combine the rinsed split peas and broth. Bring to a boil over high heat.

2. Reduce the heat to medium•low, cover, and simmer for 30•40 minutes, stirring occasionally, until the peas are very soft.

3. In a separate skillet, heat the olive oil over medium heat. Add the onion, carrots, celery, and garlic. Sauté for 5•7 minutes, until the vegetables are tender.

4. Add the sautéed vegetables to the pot with the cooked split peas. Stir in the thyme and cumin, and season with salt and pepper to taste.

5. Simmer the soup for an additional 10•15 minutes, allowing the flavors to meld. Serve the split pea and vegetable soup hot, garnished with chopped parsley if desired.

This soup is an excellent choice for a fatty liver diet for seniors for several reasons:
1. Split peas are a great source of plant•based protein, fiber, and complex carbohydrates, which can help support liver health.

2. The variety of vegetables, including carrots, celery, and onions, provide a range of vitamins, minerals, and antioxidants that can help reduce inflammation in the liver.

3. The use of low•sodium broth and the absence of heavy cream or butter make this a low•fat, low•sodium option that is suitable for seniors with fatty liver disease.

4. The simple seasoning with thyme and cumin adds flavor without the need for excessive salt.

85. Whole wheat tortilla pizza with veggies

Ingredients:

• 4 whole wheat tortillas (6•8 inches in diameter)
• 1 cup no•salt•added tomato sauce
• 1 cup shredded part•skim mozzarella cheese
• 1 cup sliced mushrooms
• 1 cup diced bell peppers (any color)
• 1/2 cup diced onions
• 1/2 cup diced zucchini
• 1 tbsp olive oil
• 1 tsp dried oregano
• Salt and pepper to taste

Instructions:

1. Preheat the oven to 400°F.

2. Brush the whole wheat tortillas lightly with olive oil on both sides. Place the tortillas on a baking sheet or pizza pan.

3. Spread the tomato sauce evenly over the tortillas, leaving a small border around the edges. Sprinkle the shredded mozzarella cheese over the sauce.

4. Top the pizzas with the sliced mushrooms, diced bell peppers, onions, and zucchini. Sprinkle the dried oregano over the vegetables and season with salt and pepper to taste.

5. Bake the pizzas for 12•15 minutes, or until the cheese is melted and the crust is lightly browned. Slice and serve the whole wheat tortilla pizzas immediately.

This dish is an excellent choice for a fatty liver diet for seniors for several reasons:

1. Whole wheat tortillas are a healthier alternative to traditional pizza crust, providing more fiber and complex carbohydrates.

2. The variety of vegetables, including mushrooms, bell peppers, onions, and zucchini, provide a range of vitamins, minerals, and antioxidants that can support liver health.

3. The use of part•skim mozzarella cheese keeps the fat content relatively low, while still providing a source of protein.

4. The simple seasoning with oregano adds flavor without the need for excessive salt, which is important for managing blood pressure and fluid retention

86. Overnight oats with peanut butter and banana

Ingredients:

• 1/2 cup old•fashioned rolled oats
• 1 cup unsweetened almond milk (or low•fat milk)
• 1 tbsp natural peanut butter
• 1 tsp honey (optional)
• 1/2 banana, sliced

Instructions:
1. In a medium•sized bowl or mason jar, combine the rolled oats and almond milk. Stir to mix well.

2. Add the peanut butter and honey (if using) and stir again until the peanut butter is evenly distributed.

3. Cover the bowl or seal the mason jar and refrigerate overnight, or for at least 6 hours.

4. In the morning, remove the overnight oats from the refrigerator and top with the sliced banana. Serve chilled or at room temperature.

This overnight oats dish is an excellent choice for a fatty liver diet for seniors for several reasons:

1. Oats are a whole grain that are high in fiber, which can help support liver health and digestion.

2. Peanut butter is a good source of healthy fats, protein, and antioxidants that can help reduce inflammation in the liver.

3. Bananas are a nutrient•dense fruit that provide potassium, fiber, and antioxidants, all of which can benefit liver function.

4. The use of unsweetened almond milk or low•fat milk keeps the dish low in saturated fat and added sugars, which are important considerations for a fatty liver diet.

5. The overnight preparation makes this a convenient and easy•to•prepare breakfast option for seniors.

87. Tofu and vegetable scramble

Ingredients:

• 1 block (14 oz) firm or extra•firm tofu, drained and crumbled
• 1 tbsp olive oil
• 1 onion, diced
• 1 bell pepper, diced
• 1 cup sliced mushrooms
• 2 cups baby spinach
• 2 cloves garlic, minced
• 1 tsp ground turmeric
• 1 tsp ground cumin
• 1/4 tsp cayenne pepper (optional)
• Salt and pepper to taste
• Chopped fresh parsley for garnish (optional)

Instructions:

1. In a large skillet, heat the olive oil over medium heat.

2. Add the diced onion, bell pepper, and sliced mushrooms. Sauté for 5•7 minutes, until the vegetables are tender.

3. Add the crumbled tofu, garlic, turmeric, cumin, and cayenne (if using) to the skillet. Stir to combine and cook for 2•3 minutes.

4. Stir in the baby spinach and cook for an additional 1•2 minutes, until the spinach is wilted.

5. Season the tofu and vegetable scramble with salt and pepper to taste. Serve the scramble hot, garnished with chopped fresh parsley if desired.

This tofu and vegetable scramble is an excellent choice for a fatty liver diet for seniors for several reasons:

1. Tofu is a plant•based protein source that is low in saturated fat, making it a great option for those with fatty liver disease.

2. The variety of vegetables, including bell peppers, mushrooms, and spinach, provide a range of vitamins, minerals, and antioxidants that can support liver health.

3. The spices, such as turmeric and cumin, have anti•inflammatory properties that can help reduce inflammation in the liver.

88. Ricotta with fresh berries and honey

Ingredients:

• 1 cup low•fat ricotta cheese
• 1 cup mixed fresh berries (such as blueberries, raspberries, and/or blackberries)
• 2 tbsp honey
• 1 tsp lemon zest (optional)

Instructions:

1. In a small bowl, scoop the ricotta cheese.

2. Top the ricotta with the mixed fresh berries.

3. Drizzle the honey over the berries and ricotta.

4. If desired, sprinkle the lemon zest over the top. Serve immediately or chill in the refrigerator until ready to serve.

This dish is an excellent choice for a fatty liver diet for seniors for several reasons:

1. Ricotta cheese is a low•fat dairy product that provides protein, calcium, and other essential nutrients.

2. Fresh berries are packed with antioxidants, fiber, and vitamins that can support liver health.

3. Honey is a natural sweetener that can provide a touch of sweetness without the need for added sugars.

4. The lemon zest (optional) adds a bright, citrusy flavor without the need for excessive salt.

The combination of protein•rich ricotta, fiber•rich berries, and a drizzle of honey creates a simple, yet satisfying dessert or snack that is both nutritious and liver•friendly.

This dish is easy to prepare, making it a convenient option for seniors who may have limited time or energy for meal preparation. It can be enjoyed on its own or paired with whole•grain crackers or a small serving of nuts for a more substantial snack.

Overall, the ricotta with fresh berries and honey is a great choice for seniors following a fatty liver diet, as it provides a balance of nutrients and flavors that can support liver health.

89. Ezekiel bread with avocado and sliced turkey

Ingredients:

- 2 slices of Ezekiel bread
- 1/2 avocado, sliced
- 3-4 slices of low-sodium, lean turkey breast
- 1 tbsp olive oil
- 1 tsp lemon juice
- Salt and pepper to taste

Instructions:

1. Toast the Ezekiel bread slices until lightly golden.

2. In a small bowl, mash the avocado slices with the olive oil and lemon juice. Season with salt and pepper.

3. Spread the mashed avocado mixture evenly over one slice of the toasted Ezekiel bread.
4. Layer the sliced turkey breast over the avocado.

5. Top with the remaining slice of Ezekiel bread. Cut the sandwich in half and serve immediately.

This Ezekiel bread sandwich with avocado and turkey is an excellent choice for a fatty liver diet for seniors for several reasons:

1. Ezekiel bread is a whole-grain, sprouted bread that is high in fiber and complex carbohydrates, which can help support liver health.

2. Avocado is a healthy source of monounsaturated fats, which can help reduce inflammation in the liver.

3. Lean turkey breast is a low-fat, high-protein option that can help maintain muscle mass and support overall health.

4. The simple seasoning with lemon juice and a small amount of olive oil provides flavor without the need for excessive salt or unhealthy fats.

The combination of whole grains, healthy fats, lean protein, and minimal added ingredients makes this Ezekiel bread sandwich a nutritious and liver-friendly choice for seniors following a fatty liver diet.

90. Tropical smoothie with spinach, pineapple, mango

Ingredients:

• 1 cup fresh spinach
• 1 cup frozen pineapple chunks
• 1 cup frozen mango chunks
• 1 cup unsweetened almond milk
• 1 tbsp ground flaxseed
• 1 tsp honey (optional)

Instructions:
1. Add all the ingredients to a high•powered blender.

2. Blend on high speed until smooth and creamy.

3. Pour into a glass and enjoy!

This smoothie is a great option for seniors on a fatty liver diet for a few reasons:

• Spinach is high in antioxidants and fiber, which can help support liver health.

• Pineapple and mango are rich in vitamins, minerals, and antioxidants that can also benefit the liver.

• Flaxseed provides healthy omega•3 fatty acids that can help reduce inflammation.

• Almond milk is a dairy•free, low•fat option that is gentle on the digestive system.

• The honey (if used) provides a touch of sweetness without spiking blood sugar levels.

This smoothie is a nutritious, delicious, and liver•friendly option for seniors. Enjoy it as a snack or light meal.

91. Roasted balsamic beets

Ingredients:

• 3 medium beets, peeled and cut into 1•inch cubes
• 2 tbsp olive oil
• 2 tbsp balsamic vinegar
• 1 tsp dried thyme
• 1/2 tsp salt
• 1/4 tsp black pepper

Instructions:
1. Preheat your oven to 400°F (200°C).

2. In a large bowl, toss the cubed beets with the olive oil, balsamic vinegar, thyme, salt, and pepper until well coated.

3. Spread the beets in a single layer on a baking sheet lined with parchment paper.

4. Roast for 25•30 minutes, stirring halfway, until the beets are tender and caramelized.

5. Serve hot or at room temperature.

This roasted balsamic beet dish is a great option for seniors on a fatty liver diet for a few reasons:

• Beets are high in antioxidants, fiber, and nutrients that can help support liver health.

• Balsamic vinegar contains polyphenols that may help reduce inflammation and improve liver function.

• The dish is low in sodium and does not contain any added sugars, making it a healthy choice.

• Roasting the beets brings out their natural sweetness, making them a tasty and satisfying side dish.

This recipe is easy to prepare and can be enjoyed as a side dish or even as a light main course. Pair it with a lean protein and a side of leafy greens for a complete and liver•friendly meal.

92. Sautéed collard greens with garlic

Ingredients:

• 1 lb collard greens, stems removed and leaves chopped
• 2 tbsp olive oil
• 3 cloves garlic, minced
• 1/4 tsp red pepper flakes (optional)
• 1/4 cup low•sodium vegetable or chicken broth
• 1 tbsp apple cider vinegar
• 1/4 tsp salt
• 1/8 tsp black pepper

Instructions:

1. In a large skillet or wok, heat the olive oil over medium heat.

2. Add the minced garlic and red pepper flakes (if using) and sauté for 1•2 minutes, until fragrant.

3. Add the chopped collard greens and sauté for 2•3 minutes, stirring frequently, until the greens start to wilt.

4. Pour in the broth and apple cider vinegar, and season with salt and pepper.

5. Reduce heat to low, cover the skillet, and let the greens simmer for 10•15 minutes, or until they are tender.

6. Remove the lid and continue cooking for 2•3 minutes, allowing any remaining liquid to evaporate. Serve hot.

This sautéed collard greens dish is a great option for seniors on a fatty liver diet for a few reasons:

• Collard greens are a nutrient•dense leafy green that is high in fiber, vitamins, and antioxidants, all of which can support liver health.
• Garlic is a natural anti•inflammatory and may help improve liver function.
• Apple cider vinegar contains acetic acid, which may help reduce fat accumulation in the liver.
• The dish is low in sodium and does not contain any added sugars or unhealthy fats.

This recipe is easy to prepare and can be enjoyed as a side dish or a light main course. Pair it with a lean protein and a whole grain for a complete and liver•friendly meal.

93. Grilled eggplant with tzatziki sauce

Ingredients:

For the Eggplant:
• 2 medium eggplants, sliced into 1/2•inch thick rounds
• 2 tbsp olive oil
• 1/2 tsp salt
• 1/4 tsp black pepper

For the Tzatziki Sauce:
• 1 cup plain Greek yogurt
• 1 cucumber, peeled, seeded, and grated
• 2 cloves garlic, minced
• 1 tbsp fresh lemon juice
• 1 tbsp chopped fresh dill
• 1/4 tsp salt
• 1/8 tsp black pepper

Instructions:
1. Preheat your grill or grill pan to medium•high heat.

2. In a large bowl, toss the eggplant slices with the olive oil, salt, and pepper until well coated.

3. Grill the eggplant slices for 3•4 minutes per side, or until they are tender and have grill marks.

4. In a medium bowl, combine all the tzatziki sauce ingredients and mix well.

5. Serve the grilled eggplant slices warm, with the tzatziki sauce on the side for dipping.

This grilled eggplant with tzatziki sauce dish is a great option for seniors on a fatty liver diet for a few reasons:

• Eggplant is a low•calorie, high•fiber vegetable that can help support liver health.
• The tzatziki sauce is made with Greek yogurt, which is a good source of protein and probiotics that can aid digestion.
• The dish is low in sodium and does not contain any added sugars or unhealthy fats.
• Grilling the eggplant adds a delicious smoky flavor without the need for additional oils or butter.

94. Quinoa with roasted vegetables

Ingredients:

• 1 cup uncooked quinoa, rinsed
• 2 cups low•sodium vegetable broth
• 1 medium zucchini, diced
• 1 medium bell pepper, diced
• 1 medium red onion, diced
• 2 cups broccoli florets
• 2 tbsp olive oil
• 1 tsp dried oregano
• 1/2 tsp garlic powder
• 1/4 tsp salt
• 1/4 tsp black pepper

Instructions:
1. Preheat your oven to 400°F (200°C).

2. In a medium saucepan, combine the quinoa and vegetable broth. Bring to a boil, then reduce heat to low, cover, and simmer for 15•20 minutes, or until the quinoa is cooked and the liquid is absorbed.

3. While the quinoa is cooking, toss the diced zucchini, bell pepper, red onion, and broccoli florets with the olive oil, oregano, garlic powder, salt, and black pepper in a large bowl.

4. Spread the seasoned vegetables on a baking sheet lined with parchment paper.

5. Roast the vegetables for 20•25 minutes, stirring halfway, until they are tender and lightly browned.

6. Fluff the cooked quinoa with a fork and transfer it to a serving bowl. Top the quinoa with the roasted vegetables and serve warm.

This quinoa with roasted vegetables dish is a great option for seniors on a fatty liver diet for a few reasons:

• Quinoa is a high•protein, high•fiber grain that can help support liver health.

• The roasted vegetables, such as zucchini, bell pepper, and broccoli, are rich in antioxidants and fiber, which can also benefit the liver.The dish is low in sodium and does not contain any added sugars or unhealthy fats.

95. Air fried jicama fries

Ingredients:

• 1 medium jicama, peeled and cut into 1/2•inch thick fry•shaped pieces
• 1 tbsp olive oil
• 1/2 tsp garlic powder
• 1/2 tsp paprika
• 1/4 tsp salt
• 1/4 tsp black pepper

Instructions:
1. Preheat your air fryer to 400°F (200°C).

2. In a large bowl, toss the jicama fries with the olive oil, garlic powder, paprika, salt, and black pepper until well coated.

3. Arrange the seasoned jicama fries in a single layer in the air fryer basket, making sure not to overcrowd.

4. Air fry for 15•20 minutes, flipping the fries halfway, until they are golden brown and crispy. Serve the air•fried jicama fries hot, as a side dish or snack.

This air•fried jicama fries recipe is a great option for seniors on a fatty liver diet for a few reasons:

• Jicama is a low•calorie, high•fiber root vegetable that can help support liver health.

• Air frying the jicama fries requires minimal oil, making them a healthier alternative to traditional deep•fried fries.

• The seasoning blend of garlic powder, paprika, salt, and pepper adds flavor without the need for unhealthy additives.

• Jicama is a good source of antioxidants and vitamins that can benefit the liver.

This recipe is easy to prepare and can be enjoyed as a side dish or a healthy snack. Pair the air•fried jicama fries with a lean protein and a side of leafy greens for a complete and liver•friendly meal.

96. Watermelon fruit salad

Ingredients:

• 4 cups cubed watermelon
• 1 cup cubed pineapple
• 1 cup blueberries
• 1 cup cubed mango
• 2 tbsp freshly squeezed lime juice
• 1 tbsp chopped fresh mint (optional)

Instructions:

1. In a large bowl, combine the cubed watermelon, pineapple, blueberries, and mango.

2. Drizzle the lime juice over the fruit and gently toss to coat.

3. If desired, sprinkle the chopped fresh mint over the top. Serve chilled or at room temperature.

This watermelon fruit salad is a great option for seniors on a fatty liver diet for a few reasons:

• Watermelon is a hydrating fruit that is low in calories and high in vitamins A and C, which can support liver health.

• Pineapple and mango are rich in antioxidants and anti•inflammatory compounds that may help reduce liver inflammation.

• Blueberries are a good source of anthocyanins, which are powerful antioxidants that can protect the liver.

• Lime juice provides a refreshing, tart flavor without the need for added sugars.

• The dish is low in sodium and does not contain any unhealthy fats.

This recipe is easy to prepare and can be enjoyed as a light, refreshing snack or a side dish. It's a great way to incorporate more nutrient•dense fruits into your diet while supporting your liver health.

97. Edamame

Ingredients:

• 1 lb frozen edamame in the pod
• 1 tbsp low•sodium soy sauce or tamari
• 1 tsp sesame oil
• 1/4 tsp sea salt (optional)

Instructions:
1. Bring a large pot of water to a boil.

2. Add the frozen edamame pods and cook for 5•7 minutes, or until the pods are tender.

3. Drain the edamame and transfer to a serving bowl.

4. Drizzle the soy sauce or tamari and sesame oil over the edamame and toss gently to coat.

5. If desired, sprinkle with a pinch of sea salt. Serve warm or at room temperature.

Edamame is an excellent choice for seniors on a fatty liver diet for several reasons:

• Edamame is a good source of plant•based protein, which can help support liver function.

• It's also high in fiber, which can help promote healthy digestion and reduce inflammation in the liver.

• Edamame contains antioxidants, such as vitamin C and isoflavones, that can help protect the liver from oxidative stress.

• The soy sauce or tamari provides a savory flavor without adding excessive sodium, while the sesame oil adds a touch of healthy fat.

• This dish is low in calories and does not contain any added sugars or unhealthy fats.

Edamame is a simple, nutritious snack or side dish that can be easily incorporated into a fatty liver•friendly diet for seniors. Enjoy it as a quick and easy way to support your liver health.

98. Three bean salad

Ingredients:

• 1 (15 oz) can low•sodium kidney beans, rinsed and drained
• 1 (15 oz) can low•sodium garbanzo beans (chickpeas), rinsed and drained
• 1 (15 oz) can low•sodium green beans, rinsed and drained
• 1/2 cup diced red onion
• 1/4 cup chopped fresh parsley
• 2 tbsp apple cider vinegar
• 1 tbsp olive oil
• 1 tsp Dijon mustard
• 1/2 tsp dried oregano
• 1/4 tsp salt
• 1/4 tsp black pepper

Instructions:
1. In a large bowl, combine the kidney beans, garbanzo beans, green beans, red onion, and parsley.

2. In a small bowl, whisk together the apple cider vinegar, olive oil, Dijon mustard, oregano, salt, and black pepper.

3. Pour the dressing over the bean mixture and toss gently to coat.

4. Cover and refrigerate for at least 30 minutes, or up to 3 days, to allow the flavors to meld. Serve chilled or at room temperature.

This three bean salad is a great option for seniors on a fatty liver diet for a few reasons:

• Beans are a good source of fiber, protein, and antioxidants, all of which can support liver health.

• The combination of different bean varieties provides a variety of nutrients and textures.

• The apple cider vinegar and Dijon mustard in the dressing provide a tangy flavor without the need for added sugars. The dish is low in sodium and does not contain any unhealthy fats.

This three bean salad is easy to prepare and can be enjoyed as a side dish or a light main course. It's a great way to incorporate more plant•based, liver•friendly foods into your diet.

99. Cucumber bites with smoked salmon

Ingredients:

- 1 English cucumber, sliced into 1/2•inch thick rounds
- 4 oz smoked salmon, cut into small pieces
- 2 tbsp plain Greek yogurt
- 1 tbsp chopped fresh dill
- 1 tsp lemon juice
- 1/4 tsp salt
- 1/8 tsp black pepper

Instructions:

1. In a small bowl, mix together the Greek yogurt, chopped dill, lemon juice, salt, and black pepper until well combined.

2. Arrange the cucumber slices on a serving platter or plate.

3. Top each cucumber slice with a small piece of smoked salmon.

4. Spoon a small amount of the yogurt•dill mixture onto each cucumber bite, spreading it evenly. Serve immediately or refrigerate until ready to serve.

This cucumber bites with smoked salmon recipe is a great option for seniors on a fatty liver diet for a few reasons:

- Cucumbers are a low•calorie, high•fiber vegetable that can help support liver health.

- Smoked salmon is a good source of omega•3 fatty acids, which can help reduce inflammation in the liver.

- Greek yogurt provides a creamy, protein•rich topping that is gentle on the digestive system.

- The fresh dill and lemon juice add flavor without the need for unhealthy additives.

- The dish is low in sodium and does not contain any added sugars or unhealthy fats.

This recipe is easy to prepare and can be enjoyed as a light snack or an appetizer. It's a great way to incorporate more nutrient•dense, liver•friendly foods into your diet.

100. Tuna stuffed tomatoes

Ingredients:

• 4 medium tomatoes, halved horizontally
• 1 (5 oz) can low•sodium tuna, drained
• 2 tbsp plain Greek yogurt
• 1 tbsp chopped fresh parsley
• 1 tsp Dijon mustard
• 1/4 tsp garlic powder
• 1/4 tsp salt
• 1/8 tsp black pepper

Instructions:

1. Preheat your oven to 375°F (190°C).

2. Scoop out the seeds and pulp from the tomato halves, leaving a small well in each half.

3. In a small bowl, mix together the tuna, Greek yogurt, parsley, Dijon mustard, garlic powder, salt, and black pepper until well combined.

4. Spoon the tuna mixture evenly into the tomato halves.

5. Arrange the stuffed tomato halves on a baking sheet or in a baking dish.

6. Bake for 15•20 minutes, or until the tomatoes are slightly softened and the tuna mixture is heated through. Serve warm or at room temperature.

This tuna stuffed tomatoes recipe is a great option for seniors on a fatty liver diet for a few reasons:

• Tomatoes are a good source of lycopene, an antioxidant that can help protect the liver.

• Tuna is a lean protein that is rich in omega•3 fatty acids, which can help reduce inflammation in the liver.

• Greek yogurt provides a creamy, protein•rich topping that is gentle on the digestive system.The dish is low in sodium and does not contain any added sugars or unhealthy fats.

This recipe is easy to prepare and can be enjoyed as a light main course or a side dish. It's a great way to incorporate more nutrient•dense, liver•friendly foods into your diet.

101. Cilantro lime shrimp

Ingredients:

- 1 lb raw shrimp, peeled and deveined
- 2 tbsp olive oil
- 2 cloves garlic, minced
- 1/4 cup chopped fresh cilantro
- 2 tbsp freshly squeezed lime juice
- 1/2 tsp ground cumin
- 1/4 tsp salt
- 1/8 tsp black pepper

Instructions:

1. In a large skillet or wok, heat the olive oil over medium•high heat.

2. Add the minced garlic and sauté for 1 minute, until fragrant.

3. Add the shrimp to the skillet and cook for 2•3 minutes per side, or until the shrimp are opaque and cooked through.

4. Remove the skillet from the heat and stir in the chopped cilantro, lime juice, cumin, salt, and black pepper.

5. Toss the shrimp to coat evenly with the cilantro•lime mixture. Serve the cilantro lime shrimp warm, over a bed of steamed quinoa or cauliflower rice.

This cilantro lime shrimp recipe is a great option for seniors on a fatty liver diet for a few reasons:

- Shrimp is a lean protein that is low in calories and high in omega•3 fatty acids, which can help reduce inflammation in the liver.

- Cilantro is a herb that contains antioxidants and may help support liver function.

- Lime juice provides a refreshing, tart flavor without the need for added sugars.

- The dish is low in sodium and does not contain any unhealthy fats.

This recipe is easy to prepare and can be enjoyed as a main course or a side dish. Pair it with a side of steamed quinoa or cauliflower rice for a complete and liver•friendly meal.

102. Butternut squash soup

Ingredients:

• 1 medium butternut squash, peeled, seeded, and cubed (about 4 cups)
• 1 medium onion, diced
• 2 cloves garlic, minced
• 4 cups low•sodium vegetable or chicken broth
• 1 tsp ground cumin
• 1/2 tsp ground cinnamon
• 1/4 tsp ground nutmeg
• 1/4 tsp salt
• 1/8 tsp black pepper
• 2 tbsp plain Greek yogurt (optional, for serving)
• 2 tbsp chopped fresh parsley (optional, for serving)

Instructions:

1. In a large pot or Dutch oven, sauté the diced onion in a small amount of olive oil over medium heat for 5•7 minutes, until translucent.

2. Add the minced garlic and sauté for an additional 1•2 minutes, until fragrant.

3. Add the cubed butternut squash, broth, cumin, cinnamon, nutmeg, salt, and black pepper. Bring the mixture to a boil.

4. Reduce the heat to low, cover the pot, and simmer for 20•25 minutes, or until the squash is very soft.

5. Using an immersion blender or a regular blender, puree the soup until smooth and creamy.

6. Serve the butternut squash soup warm, with a dollop of plain Greek yogurt and a sprinkle of chopped fresh parsley, if desired.

This butternut squash soup is a great option for seniors on a fatty liver diet for a few reasons:

• Butternut squash is a nutrient•dense vegetable that is high in fiber, vitamins, and antioxidants, all of which can support liver health.

• The spices, such as cumin, cinnamon, and nutmeg, add flavor without the need for unhealthy additives.

103. Chickpea and farro salad

Ingredients:

• 1 cup dry farro, cooked according to package instructions
• 1 (15 oz) can low•sodium chickpeas, rinsed and drained
• 1 cup diced cucumber
• 1/2 cup diced red bell pepper
• 1/4 cup diced red onion
• 2 tbsp chopped fresh parsley
• 2 tbsp olive oil
• 2 tbsp red wine vinegar
• 1 tsp Dijon mustard
• 1/2 tsp dried oregano
• 1/4 tsp salt
• 1/8 tsp black pepper

Instructions:
1. In a large bowl, combine the cooked farro, chickpeas, diced cucumber, red bell pepper, red onion, and chopped parsley.

2. In a small bowl, whisk together the olive oil, red wine vinegar, Dijon mustard, dried oregano, salt, and black pepper.

3. Pour the dressing over the farro and chickpea mixture and toss gently to coat.

4. Cover and refrigerate the salad for at least 30 minutes, or up to 3 days, to allow the flavors to meld. Serve chilled or at room temperature.

This chickpea and farro salad is a great option for seniors on a fatty liver diet for a few reasons:

• Chickpeas are a good source of plant•based protein, fiber, and antioxidants that can support liver health.

• Farro is a whole grain that is high in fiber and nutrients, which can also benefit the liver.
• The vegetables, such as cucumber and bell pepper, provide additional vitamins, minerals, and fiber.

• The olive oil and red wine vinegar dressing adds healthy fats and a tangy flavor without the need for unhealthy additives.

• The dish is low in sodium and does not contain any added sugars.

104. Chicken lettuce wraps

Ingredients:

• 1 lb ground chicken or turkey
• 1 tbsp sesame oil
• 2 cloves garlic, minced
• 1 tbsp grated fresh ginger
• 2 tbsp low•sodium soy sauce or tamari
• 1 tbsp rice vinegar
• 1 tsp honey
• 1/4 tsp red pepper flakes (optional)
• 1 cup shredded carrots
• 1/2 cup diced water chestnuts
• 1/4 cup chopped green onions
• 12•16 large lettuce leaves (such as romaine or bibb)

Instructions:
1. In a large skillet or wok, cook the ground chicken or turkey over medium•high heat, breaking it up with a wooden spoon, until it's no longer pink, about 5•7 minutes.

2. Drain any excess fat from the skillet.

3. Add the sesame oil, minced garlic, and grated ginger to the skillet. Sauté for 1•2 minutes, until fragrant.

4. Stir in the soy sauce or tamari, rice vinegar, honey, and red pepper flakes (if using). Simmer for 2•3 minutes, until the sauce has thickened slightly.

5. Remove the skillet from the heat and stir in the shredded carrots, diced water chestnuts, and chopped green onions. To serve, spoon the chicken mixture into the lettuce leaves and enjoy.

These chicken lettuce wraps are a great option for seniors on a fatty liver diet for a few reasons:

• Ground chicken or turkey is a lean protein that is low in fat and calories.
• The vegetables, such as carrots and water chestnuts, provide fiber and antioxidants that can support liver health.
• The soy sauce or tamari, rice vinegar, and honey provide flavor without the need for excessive sodium or added sugars.
• Lettuce leaves are a low•calorie, nutrient•dense alternative to traditional wraps or buns.
• The dish is easy to prepare and can be enjoyed as a light main course or a snack.

105. Twice baked potatoes with broccoli

Ingredients:

- 4 medium russet potatoes
- 1 cup steamed broccoli florets, chopped
- 1/2 cup plain Greek yogurt
- 1/4 cup low•fat milk
- 2 tbsp grated Parmesan cheese
- 1 tsp garlic powder
- 1/2 tsp salt
- 1/4 tsp black pepper

Instructions:

1. Preheat your oven to 400°F (200°C).

2. Bake the potatoes directly on the oven rack for 50•60 minutes, or until they are tender when pierced with a fork.

3. Allow the potatoes to cool for 10 minutes, then cut them in half lengthwise.

4. Scoop the potato flesh into a medium bowl, leaving a thin layer of potato in the skins.

5. Add the steamed and chopped broccoli, Greek yogurt, milk, Parmesan cheese, garlic powder, salt, and black pepper to the bowl. Mash and mix until well combined.

6. Spoon the potato•broccoli mixture back into the potato skins, dividing it evenly.

7. Place the stuffed potato halves on a baking sheet and bake for an additional 15•20 minutes, or until heated through and lightly browned on top. Serve hot.

This twice•baked potato recipe with broccoli is a great option for seniors on a fatty liver diet for a few reasons:

- Potatoes are a good source of complex carbohydrates, fiber, and potassium, which can support liver health.
- Broccoli is a nutrient•dense vegetable that is high in antioxidants and fiber, both of which can benefit the liver.
- Greek yogurt provides a creamy, protein•rich topping that is gentle on the digestive system.
- The dish is low in sodium and does not contain any unhealthy fats or added sugars.

106. Coconut lime baked cod

Ingredients:

• 1 lb cod fillets, cut into 4 portions
• 1/4 cup unsweetened coconut milk
• 2 tbsp freshly squeezed lime juice
• 1 tsp grated lime zest
• 1 tsp honey
• 1/4 tsp ground cumin
• 1/4 tsp salt
• 1/8 tsp black pepper

Instructions:

1. Preheat your oven to 400°F (200°C).

2. In a small bowl, whisk together the coconut milk, lime juice, lime zest, honey, cumin, salt, and black pepper.

3. Place the cod fillets in a baking dish and pour the coconut lime mixture over the top, making sure the fish is evenly coated.

4. Bake for 15•20 minutes, or until the cod is opaque and flakes easily with a fork.

5. Serve the coconut lime baked cod warm, garnished with additional lime zest or chopped fresh cilantro, if desired.

This coconut lime baked cod recipe is a great option for seniors on a fatty liver diet for a few reasons:

• Cod is a lean, low•fat fish that is high in protein and omega•3 fatty acids, which can help reduce inflammation in the liver.

• Coconut milk provides a creamy, dairy•free sauce that is gentle on the digestive system.

• Lime juice and zest add a refreshing, tart flavor without the need for added sugars.

• The dish is low in sodium and does not contain any unhealthy fats.

This recipe is easy to prepare and can be enjoyed as a main course or a light meal. Serve it with a side of roasted vegetables or a fresh salad for a complete and liver•friendly meal.

107. Cauliflower fried rice

Ingredients:

- 1 head of cauliflower, cut into florets
- 1 tbsp sesame oil
- 1 cup diced onion
- 1 cup diced carrots
- 1 cup frozen peas
- 2 cloves garlic, minced
- 2 tbsp low•sodium soy sauce or tamari
- 1 tsp grated fresh ginger
- 1/4 tsp ground white pepper
- 2 eggs, lightly beaten (optional)
- 2 tbsp chopped fresh cilantro (optional)

Instructions:

1. In a food processor, pulse the cauliflower florets until they resemble the size and texture of rice grains. Set aside.

2. In a large skillet or wok, heat the sesame oil over medium•high heat. Add the diced onion and carrots and sauté for 3•4 minutes, until they start to soften.

3. Add the frozen peas, minced garlic, and grated ginger. Sauté for an additional 2 minutes.

4. Add the riced cauliflower to the skillet and stir to combine. Sauté for 5•7 minutes, until the cauliflower is tender. Drizzle the soy sauce or tamari over the cauliflower mixture and stir to coat.

5. If using, push the cauliflower mixture to the sides of the skillet and pour the beaten eggs into the center. Scramble the eggs, then mix them into the cauliflower.

6. Remove the skillet from the heat and stir in the ground white pepper. Garnish the cauliflower fried rice with chopped fresh cilantro, if desired. Serve hot.

This cauliflower fried rice recipe is a great option for seniors on a fatty liver diet for a few reasons:

- Cauliflower is a low•carb, nutrient•dense vegetable that can help support liver health.

- The dish is low in sodium and does not contain any unhealthy fats or added sugars.

108. Minestrone soup

Ingredients:

• 2 tbsp olive oil
• 1 onion, diced
• 3 cloves garlic, minced
• 2 carrots, peeled and diced
• 2 celery stalks, diced
• 1 zucchini, diced
• 1 (15 oz) can low•sodium diced tomatoes
• 4 cups low•sodium vegetable or chicken broth
• 1 (15 oz) can low•sodium kidney beans, rinsed and drained
• 1 (15 oz) can low•sodium cannellini beans, rinsed and drained
• 1 cup small whole•wheat pasta (such as ditalini or elbow macaroni)
• 2 tsp dried oregano
• 1 tsp dried basil
• 1/4 tsp red pepper flakes (optional)
• Salt and black pepper to taste
• 2 cups chopped kale or spinach (optional)
• 2 tbsp grated Parmesan cheese (optional)

Instructions:

1. In a large pot or Dutch oven, heat the olive oil over medium heat.

2. Add the diced onion and sauté for 3•4 minutes, until translucent.

3. Add the minced garlic and sauté for an additional 1 minute.

4. Stir in the diced carrots, celery, and zucchini. Sauté for 5•7 minutes, until the vegetables start to soften.

5. Add the diced tomatoes, vegetable or chicken broth, kidney beans, cannellini beans, whole•wheat pasta, oregano, basil, and red pepper flakes (if using). Season with salt and black pepper to taste.

6. Bring the soup to a boil, then reduce the heat and simmer for 15•20 minutes, or until the pasta is tender.

7. If using, stir in the chopped kale or spinach and cook for an additional 2•3 minutes, until the greens are wilted. Serve the minestrone soup hot, garnished with grated Parmesan cheese, if desired.

109. Vegetable whole wheat flatbread pizza

Ingredients:

For the Flatbread:
• 1 cup whole wheat flour
• 1/2 cup all•purpose flour
• 1 tsp baking powder
• 1/4 tsp salt
• 1/2 cup plain Greek yogurt
• 2 tbsp water

For the Toppings:
• 1 cup sliced mushrooms
• 1 cup diced bell peppers
• 1 cup diced zucchini
• 1/2 cup diced red onion
• 1 cup low•sodium tomato sauce
• 1/2 cup shredded part•skim mozzarella cheese

Instructions:
1. Preheat your oven to 400°F (200°C).

2. In a medium bowl, whisk together the whole wheat flour, all•purpose flour, baking powder, and salt.

3. Add the Greek yogurt and water, and stir until a dough forms. Knead the dough briefly on a lightly floured surface.

4. Roll or stretch the dough into a thin, rectangular flatbread shape and place it on a baking sheet lined with parchment paper.

5. Bake the flatbread for 10•12 minutes, or until lightly golden.

6. Remove the flatbread from the oven and top it with the sliced mushrooms, diced bell peppers, zucchini, and red onion.

7. Spread the tomato sauce evenly over the vegetables and sprinkle the shredded mozzarella cheese on top.

8. Return the pizza to the oven and bake for an additional 10•12 minutes, or until the cheese is melted and bubbly. Slice and serve the vegetable whole wheat flatbread pizza hot.

110. Mango chia pudding

Ingredients:

• 1 cup unsweetened almond milk
• 1/4 cup chia seeds
• 1 ripe mango, peeled and diced (about 1 cup)
• 1 tbsp honey (optional)
• 1/2 tsp vanilla extract
• 1/4 tsp ground cinnamon

Instructions:

1. In a medium bowl, whisk together the almond milk and chia seeds. Cover and refrigerate for at least 2 hours, or up to 24 hours, stirring occasionally, until the chia seeds have thickened the mixture into a pudding•like consistency.

2. Once the chia pudding has set, stir in the diced mango, honey (if using), vanilla extract, and ground cinnamon until well combined.

3. Divide the mango chia pudding evenly into 4 serving bowls or jars.

4. Refrigerate the pudding for an additional 30 minutes to 1 hour before serving, to allow the flavors to meld. Serve chilled.

This mango chia pudding is a great option for seniors on a fatty liver diet for a few reasons:

• Chia seeds are a good source of fiber, protein, and omega•3 fatty acids, all of which can support liver health.

• Mangoes are a nutrient•dense fruit that are high in vitamins, minerals, and antioxidants, which can also benefit the liver.

• The almond milk provides a dairy•free, low•fat base that is gentle on the digestive system.

• The honey (if used) provides a touch of sweetness without spiking blood sugar levels.The dish is low in sodium and does not contain any unhealthy fats.

This mango chia pudding is a refreshing, nutrient•dense dessert or snack that can be easily incorporated into a fatty liver•friendly diet for seniors. Enjoy it as a healthy treat that supports your liver health.

*Thank you for joining us on this culinary journey through the **"Fatty Liver Diet Cookbook for Seniors: 110+ Nourishing and Satisfying Meals for Optimal Liver Health."** We hope this collection of recipes has inspired you to embrace a healthier lifestyle and provided you with the tools to support your liver health.*

Maintaining liver health is crucial for overall well-being, especially as we age. By choosing the right foods, you can make a significant impact on your liver function and general health. This cookbook was designed with your needs in mind, offering delicious, easy-to-prepare meals that cater to the nutritional requirements of seniors. Each recipe is a step towards better health, combining taste and nutrition to ensure that healthy eating is a pleasure, not a chore.

As you continue your journey towards optimal liver health, remember that consistency is key. Incorporating these liver-friendly recipes into your daily routine can lead to lasting health benefits. Pairing a balanced diet with regular physical activity, adequate hydration, and sufficient rest will further enhance your overall health and well-being.

Beyond the recipes, we hope you've found the meal planning tips, nutritional information, and shopping advice useful. These tools are designed to empower you to make informed decisions about your diet and lifestyle, ensuring that you can sustain these healthy habits long-term.

We encourage you to share these recipes with friends and family, spreading the joy of healthy eating and supporting those around you in their health journeys. Cooking and eating together can be a wonderful way to connect and enjoy life's simple pleasures.

In closing, we wish you continued success in your pursuit of a healthier liver and a happier life. May these recipes nourish not only your body but also your spirit, bringing joy and vitality to your days.

Here's to your health, happiness, and many delicious meals ahead!

Happy cooking, and take care.

9 798328 008426